BASICS OF MAGNETIC RESONANCE IMAGING

TOPICS IN NEUROLOGY

BASICS OF MAGNETIC RESONANCE IMAGING

by

WILLIAM OLDENDORF, M.D.

and

WILLIAM OLDENDORF, JR.

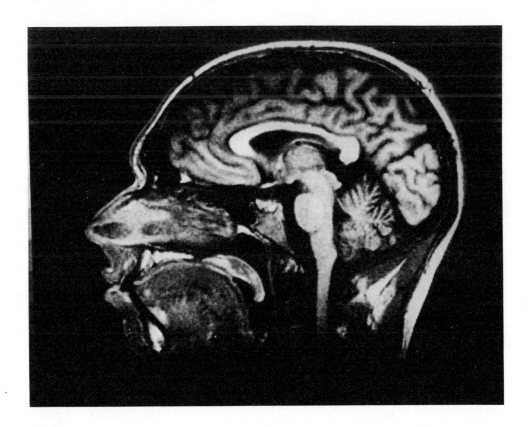

MARTINUS NIJHOFF PUBLISHING
A MEMBER OF THE KLUWER ACADEMIC PUBLISHERS GROUP
BOSTON/DORDRECHT/LANCASTER

Distributors

for the United States and Canada: Kluwer Academic Publishers, 101 Philip Drive Assinippi Park, Norwell, MA, 02061, USA

for the UK and Ireland: Kluwer Academic Publishers, MTP Press Limited, Falcon House, Queen Square, Lancaster LA1 1RN, UNITED KINGDOM

for all other countries: Kluwer Academic Publishers Group, Distribution Centre, P.O. Box 322, 3300 AH Dordrecht, THE NETHERLANDS

Frontispiece: from GE Medical Systems

Library of Congress Cataloging in Publication Data

Oldendorf, William H.
  Basics of magnetic resonance imaging.

  (Topics in neurology)
  Bibliography: p.
  Includes index.
  1. Magnetic resonance imaging. I. Oldendorf, William.
II. Title. III. Series.
RC78.7.N83043 1987   616.07'57   87–20424
ISBN 0-89838-964-X

Dedicated, to Stella Z.

CONTENTS

ACKNOWLEDGEMENTS

Writing an introductory text about a complex subject is a difficult task which would not have been possible without the help of two people:

The first of these is Leon D. Braun, the artist who produced the many detailed illustrations which accompany the text. The second is Nancy Goldsmith-Rose, whose knowledge of both science and language helped clarify the presentation of the text.

Many colleagues have generously offered their time to answer questions. The authors are especially indebted to Dr. Ray Gangarosa (Picker International), Dr. Frank Anet, Dr. Donald Fredkin, and Dr. William G. Bradley.

As always, many thanks to Stella Z. Oldendorf, for many long hours of material assistance and moral support.

PREFACE

This book is not intended as a general text on MRI. It is written as an introduction to the field, for nonexperts. We present here a simple exposition of certain aspects of MRI that are important to understand to use this valuable diagnostic tool intelligently in a clinical setting. The basic principles are presented nonmathematically, using no equations and a minimum of symbols and abbreviations. For those requiring a deeper understanding of MRI, this book will help facilitate the transition to standard texts.

Chapters 1 through 4 provide a general introduction to the phenomenon of nuclear magnetic resonance and how it is used in imaging. Chapter 1 discusses magnetic resonance, using a compass needle as an example. In Chapter 2, the transition to the magnetic resonance of the atomic nucleus is made. Chapter 3 describes the principles of imaging. In Chapter 4, the terms T_1 and T_2 are described and their relationship to tissue characterization; the fundamental role of thermal magnetic noise in T_1 and T_2 is discussed.

Chapter 5 introduces the magnetization vector as a convenient means of expressing nuclear behavior. T_1 and T_2 are described in more depth, and their role in imaging presented. The spin-echo pulse sequence and the relationships of T_1 and T_2 to image brightness are introduced. This complex chapter is not necessary for an understanding of the remainder of the book; the reader can proceed from Chapter 4 directly to Chapter 6.

Chapter 6 describes the basic hardware components of an MRI scanner, including the design of the main magnet and gradient coils.

Chapters 7 and 8 review X-ray computerized tomography (CT) and its relationship to MRI. Limitations and advantages of each imaging technique are discussed. Some clinical correlates of relaxation processes (T_1 and T_2) are presented.

Chapter 9 speculates on future directions of this versatile clinical probe.

The appendix provides a brief introduction to the quantum processes in MRI.

A NOTE ON SYMBOLS AND ABBREVIATIONS

The physical process upon which MRI is based — nuclear magnetic resonance (NMR) — was recognized in 1946. For the next 30 years it was used largely as a chemical analytical tool under the name NMR. Consequently, the first scanners to exploit nuclear magnetic resonance to produce medical images were termed *NMR scanners*.

However, the use of the word *nuclear* caused concern among patients, who associated nuclear with radioactive, although there is no radioactivity or indeed any ionizing radiation involved. As a result, the term *MRI* came into use, although some confusion still exists about the use of these terms. In this book, *NMR* refers to the basic phenomenon of nuclear magnetic resonance (and to its use in chemical analysis in a laboratory setting); *MRI* refers to the process that exploits the physical phenomenon to make medical images in a clinical setting.

The basic physical phenomenon of NMR is easily demonstrated, but its application to MRI is more complex; although the crude phenomenon can be detected with very simple equipment, to fully exploit its many ramifications requires an elaborate theory and complicated equipment.

As in most scientific specialties, the traditional NMR literature assigns many abbreviations or symbols to various aspects of the process. An excellent book published in 1971 (Farrar and Becker) lists 127 such abbreviations. Although many of these represent simple units, most refer to complex phenomena. To aid the reader's introduction to this field, we have used a nonmathematical approach and have chosen to use no symbols or abbreviations, except: CT, NMR, MRI, T_1, and T_2.

BASICS OF MAGNETIC RESONANCE IMAGING

INTRODUCTION: DIAGNOSTIC PROBES

The physician confronted by a sick patient needs to know the nature of the malfunction and often is starved for information that might lead to a diagnosis. Our vision sees only the surface. What we wish to examine is the body's interior. To provide this information, the patient's body is interrogated by means of various probes. Each probe interacts in some way with the tissues. The nature and extent of the interaction and its anatomic location are noted.

Classical physical diagnosis is the art of using little or no artificial apparatus to learn about the properties of living tissue. It uses the simplest probe — the palpating finger — which moves over the surface of the patient, interrogating such features as skin textures or subsurface masses. Limited access to the inside of the body may be gained through examination of its orifices, but this provides information only about nearby structures. Using only touch and position senses, the physician performs the simplest form of clinical image reconstruction: imagination. The sensory input from the fingers is used to form an image in the mind of the nature of the interior of the body. The physician's imagination, enriched by past training and experience, makes this technique surprisingly accurate. An examination of the abdomen by a skilled surgeon feeling for internal organs and listening to their sounds can produce a remarkably informative image of the unseen abdominal organs.

In modern terms, the physician is using a sequence of instructions (a mental algorithm) by which the image is constructed in the mind from the simple palpation (input data). Although the probe needed for imaging by palpation is inexpensive and completely portable, the technique provides only very limited information and for only a few accessible anatomical regions.

In another of the common probing procedures, percussion, the fingers of one hand are placed on the surface of the body and the fingers of the other hand are struck against them creating a new probe, the advancing compression wave front (sound) which passes into the body. Over the chest, a certain quality of thump is heard and over the abdomen another. The character of the sound is determined by the shape and size of gas-filled cavities in the chest or intestine. Audible resonances in the gas in these regions are evoked by input of sound energy, and they are heard and interpreted by the physician. Knowing the general internal anatomy and what commonly goes wrong, a crude image of likely internal abnormalities forms in the physician's mind.

In magnetic resonance imaging (MRI) an analogous process of percussion is carried out. Instead of being percussed for audible resonances in gas-filled cavities, the body is percussed magnetically and listened to for magnetic resonances, which are then analyzed.

MRI can be thought of as magnetic percussion. While simple manual percussion can provide only very limited information about the tissues, it can often be of use in patient management. Its limited information value is balanced by its great simplicity and by the absence of any apparatus other than the physician's hands (the transmitter), ears (the receiver), and brain (the computer), which together serve to construct an image of the body's internal condition.

MODERN PROBES

Much of the progress in diagnostic research has been directed at the development of more versatile probes. The first of these probes was the X-ray, discovered by Roentgen in 1895. To varying degrees, X-rays penetrate all visually opaque objects; their freedom of passage varies according to the nature of the object.

Roentgen's first subject was a hand, which he placed over a photographic plate so that the X-rays cast a shadow of its bones. Because the X-rays from early sources were very weak (by modern standards), they could penetrate only a short distance through tissues; as a consequence, the relatively thin hand was a favorite early subject for demonstration.

Roentgen provided the physician with access to the interior of the living body, beyond the reach of existing probes. It was nearly as revolutionary as the first anatomical dissection had been, several centuries earlier.

Although they are enormously valuable, there is evidence of an impending decline in the use of X-rays in clinical diagnosis. Newer probes which are more informative are appearing. Just as palpation is useful but limited in scope, simple shadow images using X-rays are useful but are unable to provide direct images of the soft tissues, where most disease arises.

THE INTRODUCTION OF CT

Until 1972, ordinary medical radiographic films were made using essentially the same apparatus and techniques of a half-century earlier. In 1972, EMI Ltd. of England made public the prototype of an apparatus that has been recognized as the most significant development in clinical use of X-rays since their discovery by Roentgen — the computerized tomographic (CT) scanner.

This new development was a complete departure from classical radiography, which had used a wide shower of X-rays to cast shadows of body parts on a photographic film. In 1967, Godfrey N. Hounsfield, an EMI computer engineer, began applying a computer to the problem of reconstructing cross-sectional images of the body from information gathered by a narrow beam of X-rays. The beam entered the edge of the cross-section of the body being imaged. After traversing the body, the emerging X-rays were counted and the number lost in passage through the body calculated. The position of the beam was changed many times in the course of the scan so that any one cross-section of the body was examined many times from many directions. A computer, properly instructed, reconstructed the density (specific gravity) of the tissue in the cross-section being examined.

The resulting CT scan could be thought of as though the cross-section had been cut from the body, placed on a radiographic plate, exposed, and the resulting film developed and viewed on a view-box much as an ordinary radiograph (Figure 1).

CT and related diagnostic imaging methods provide so much three-dimensional structural detail that displaying the body's interior as viewed

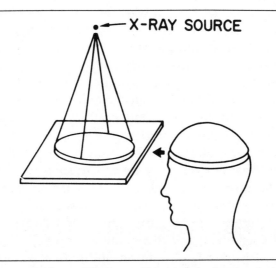

Figure 1. An image comparable to a CT scan could be made by freezing the body, sawing out a slab of tissue, placing the slab on an X-ray plate, and making a radiograph of it. CT accomplishes the same process using a beam of X-rays, which enters the slice from its edge and traverses the entire slice. The image is then reconstructed by a computer.

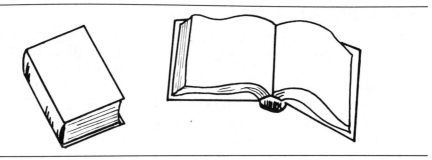

Figure 2. A closed book could not be read, even if the pages and cover were transparent, because the words would all be superimposed. Opening the book isolates a page, allowing its detail to be seen. This is equivalent to performing tomography. The wealth of detail provided by modern imaging techniques requires the image to be displayed tomographically.

from an external point (as in standard radiography) causes the structures to be superimposed on each other. It is as though one were attempting to examine the contents of a book that had been specially constructed with transparent cover and pages, so that only the type was visible. With the book closed, the words and letters of the text would be superimposed and, even if the book were just a few pages thick, only a meaningless jumble would be visible. The solution is to open the book and look at one page at a time. Each time we open a book and view the exposed pages individually, we perform tomography on the book (Figure 2). Similarly, in the body, we must slice it up (perform tomography) and look at one slice at a time.

CT scanning was immediately recognized as revolutionary, and subsequent experience has amply confirmed this first impression. The earliest images, which were exclusively of brain, were crude by modern standards but showed pathology clearly enough to predict that CT would be a quantum leap forward in medical diagnosis. Among many other honors, Hounsfield received the Nobel prize for this work in 1979.

CT scanning allowed, during life, a limited but repeatable view of brain structure that had previously been available only after death, when the brain could be removed from the head and chemically fixed to make it firm enough to be cut mechanically into sections. CT allowed what was, in essence, a limited autopsy during life. Because it was painless and harmless, CT could be employed at even the faintest suspicion of early brain disease. And, unlike the diagnostic tests available up to that time, it could be repeated freely to follow the course of a disease. As a result, many nonfatal diseases were accessible to scrutiny for the first time. Fatal diseases were visualized throughout their course and not just at their terminal stage. Although we emphasize the head in this book, almost any region of the body could be used as an example.

X-ray CT has become as vital to the practice of neurology and neurosurgery as radiography of the skeleton is to orthopedic surgery. Our knowledge of cerebrovascular disease has been greatly advanced and many traditional beliefs, which were based on observation of the clinical course and subsequent autopsy (perhaps years after the disease began), have been completely changed. Management of brain tumors has been greatly facilitated by their being recognized accurately at much earlier stages of development. The acute management of head trauma has been greatly advanced. Brain atrophy in many degenerative diseases can now be measured harmlessly and more accurately than at autopsy. In many elderly patients, considerable atrophy is seen, often without significant brain dysfunction.

Many other examples could be given of the major impact CT scanning has had on diagnostic medicine, but its effect can be summed up as revolutionary. By 1985 there were approximately 7000 CT scanners worldwide, about one third each in Japan and the United States, and the remaining one third in other countries.

With this resounding success story, why is CT application levelling off? Development of newer, advanced CT scanners has nearly ceased and sales are levelling off, mostly to replace older scanners that are no longer state-of-the-art.

Part of the reason for its decline is the limited tissue characterization offered by CT. Because the extent to which X-rays interact with tissue is proportional to the density of tissue, a CT scan is a map of specific gravity. With injection of contrast media, we see a superimposed distribution of iodine. These two sources of information are all that are offered by CT scanning (see Chapter 7).

Much of the decline in interest in CT scanning is due to the appearance of a much more sophisticated diagnostic probe: the magnetic field.

MAGNETIC PROBE

The subject of this book is magnetic resonance imaging (MRI), the technology that utilizes this highly versatile new probe. The interaction of magnetic fields and tissue atoms is so elaborate that much more information can be obtained than with X-rays. New strategies are constantly being developed so that tissue characterization has improved dramatically over the past few years, and there is every reason to believe that the field will continue to develop for many years to come.

Just as there are many more moves and strategies in the game of chess than there are in checkers, the tissue interaction available in MRI potentially offers very much more tissue characterization than is possible with CT.

THE DECLINING AUTOPSY

There have been so many advances in clinical imaging techniques in recent years that the postmortem examination is becoming obsolete. This is not in itself a cause for concern, however, since it should be the indirect purpose of all diagnostic research to make the traditional autopsy unnecessary. During the past century, the autopsy has been considered the ultimate standard of diagnosis. This remains true today, but the role of the autopsy is waning. In major teaching centers, only about one third as many autopsies are performed as two decades ago. There are several factors contributing to this, such as the desire for cost containment and the refusal of most health insurance companies to pay for them.

But a major factor is that few "curiosity" autopsies are now performed. Before modern imaging, patients often died without a clear diagnosis ever having been made; the cause of death was clarified only at autopsy. With modern diagnostic methods, this happens much less often, and a plausible diagnosis is usually arrived at during life. Modern imaging methods play a large role in arriving at this diagnosis.

Although the autopsy is a superb diagnostic and teaching process, it has severe limitations and disadvantages. First of all, the person being autopsied cannot benefit from the procedure. Usually, only fatal disease processes are seen, and only in their terminal state; nonfatal diseases are seen only coincidentally. Since the autopsy may be performed several days after death, postmortem artifacts are prominent; these are superimposed on the often prolonged dying process, which may have created its own artifacts. The results of the autopsy are largely anatomical; only limited chemical studies are possible. The disturbances in function which were the source of patient complaints during life may only be inferred.

X-ray computerized tomography (CT) did much to improve the accuracy of clinical diagnosis, but its limitations are now being realized. MRI supplies a wealth of information, exceeding CT in most instances. It promises a giant step toward the premortem autopsy which we so urgently seek since, while there is life, there is hope of benefitting the patient under study.

Still, the autopsy will not disappear for a very long time. So much information has been accumulated by pathologists that the vast data bank of traditional histology will remain the gold standard for many decades to come.

CHAPTER 1: MAGNETIC RESONANCE: A FAMILIAR EXAMPLE

Magnetic resonance is an interaction between a magnet and a magnetic field. The most familiar magnet is a compass needle. The most familiar magnetic field is that of the Earth. The most familiar interaction of a magnet with a magnetic field is the alignment of a compass needle with the Earth's field: The compass points north and south.

If we start with a compass needle at rest, pointing north, and then tap the tip of the needle with our finger, the needle deflects away from north but is then drawn back toward its original northerly orientation. It overshoots north and starts a to-and-fro oscillatory movement, which continues until all of the energy the needle absorbed from our finger is lost to mechanical friction and air drag. The compass again comes to rest pointing north (Figure 3).

The frequency of this oscillatory movement is the needle's *natural frequency*, which depends both on the characteristics of the compass needle — its dimensions, strength of magnetization, and weight — and on the strength of the external field. This last point is worth repeating: The natural frequency is proportional to the external field strength. In a stronger magnetic field, the compass needle oscillates faster; if the external field strength doubles, the natural frequency doubles.

The magnetic field of the Earth is not uniform over its entire surface. The field converges at the north and south magnetic poles and spreads out over the surface of the Earth in between. Near the poles the Earth's field is

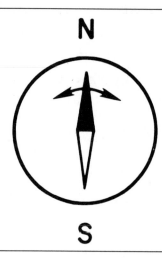

Figure 3. A compass needle aligns itself north and south in the Earth's magnetic field. If deflected from its north-south heading, it oscillates at a frequency proportional to the local magnetic field strength.

strongest, being about 0.7 gauss (the gauss is a common unit of magnetic field strength) and at the equator weakest, about 0.3 gauss. Between the equator and poles, there is a gradual transition in field strength (Figure 4A).

Such a gradual change in field strength between one location and another is called a *magnetic field gradient*, or simply a *gradient*, a term to be much used later in this book.

We could construct a compass that oscillates at a natural frequency of one cycle per second at the equator. If we travelled north with the compass, we would find the frequency of oscillation changing gradually: the farther north, the higher the frequency of oscillation. At the north pole, the compass would oscillate about 2.3 cycles per second because the Earth's field is 2.3 times stronger there. If properly calibrated, the compass needle could be used as a crude navigational device using natural frequency to estimate latitude. (Figure 4B).

In this simple example, we have the essential elements of MRI:

1. A compass needle, when placed in a magnetic field, aligns itself with the field.
2. When stimulated, the compass needle oscillates at a frequency proportional to the strength of the magnetic field.
3. In a gradient magnetic field that varies in strength in a known manner, the location of the compass needle can be deduced from its frequency of oscillation.

We further note that this process includes a means of stimulation (our finger) and a means of detecting the movement (our eye).

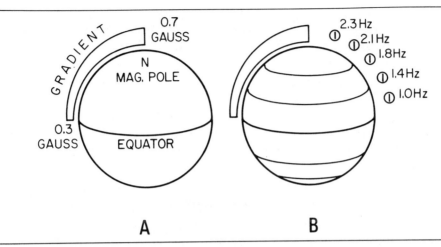

Figure 4A + B. (A) The Earth's magnetic field is not uniform. Since it converges on the poles, the field strength there is greater than at the equator. The gradually rising field strength between equator and poles constitutes a magnetic field gradient.
(B) A compass oscillates faster near the pole. Properly calibrated, it could be used as a crude navigational device, to determine latitude from frequency of oscillation.

ALTERNATIVE MEANS OF STIMULATION AND DETECTION

We could also develop means of stimulating the compass needle and observing its subsequent behavior other than simply tapping it with our finger and watching the movement.

Detection

We can, of course, observe the movement of the compass needle visually, but if we were unable to do this and needed to instrument this navigational device electronically, we could easily do so.

The simplest means of measuring the oscillatory movement of the compass needle after stimulation would be to place near it a coil of wire which would act as an antenna. Since the needle is itself a magnet, its movement would induce voltage in the coil. Its oscillatory frequency could be determined if the induced voltage were amplified and sent to an electronic frequency analyzer. By this means, a simple number (its frequency) could indicate the latitude of the compass without the compass actually being seen.

Stimulation

If instead of applying a single strong tap we applied an evenly spaced series of very light taps, we would find, upon varying the frequency of the tapping, that the excursion of the needle would change. At one particular frequency, a maximum excursion would be noted. This would be at the natural or resonant frequency.

A familiar example of applying energy at a particular frequency is pushing a child on a playground swing. After a single push, the swing moves to-and-fro at its natural frequency. We intuitively time our series of pushes to correspond to this frequency. Like the compass needle, the swing can most efficiently absorb the energy of our push at this, its resonant frequency. Attempting to push at other frequencies would be less efficient.

If we wished to remotely stimulate the compass needle, rather than tap it, we could place a small coil of wire adjacent to one end. Passing brief pulses of current through this coil creates a fluctuating magnetic field proportional to the current, thus imparting brief magnetic kicks to the needle. If we varied the frequency of the pulses, at one frequency the resulting amplitude of swing would be greatest. This is the resonant frequency, the impulse rate at which the needle absorbs energy most efficiently.

This is the phenomenon of resonance: The most efficient absorption of energy occurs at the needle's natural, or resonant, frequency. Stimulating it at higher or lower frequencies results in lesser amplitudes of swing.

Resonance is the result of a set of conditions in which an object can most efficiently absorb energy from an alternating source. In the case of a compass needle, the resonant frequency is determined by the length and mass of the needle, how strongly magnetized it is, and the strength of the external field it is in. The phenomenon of resonance pervades science. It governs the exchange of energy between fingers and guitar strings, between earthquake shocks and buildings, between passing trains and rattling windows, between wind and swaying bridges, and even between atomic nuclei.

CHAPTER 2: NUCLEAR MAGNETIC RESONANCE

The behavior of compass needles in the Earth's magnetic field was introduced in Chapter 1 to present the concept of magnetic resonance. A compass needle is actually a small bar magnet which oscillates at a particular frequency when driven from its resting state. The frequency of its oscillation is proportional to the field strength in which it finds itself. While the simplest means of stimulating a compass needle is by a simple tap of the finger, it can also be driven from its resting state by subjecting it to an alternating external magnetic field. When the alternation occurs at the needle's natural or resonant frequency, the compass needle absorbs energy.

We are interested in the magnetic properties of living tissues, which contain no compass needles. But there are small magnets with some of the properties of a compass needle: the nuclei of certain atoms.

MAGNETIC NUCLEI

Among the elements with magnetic nuclei, hydrogen is of the greatest biological interest, both because it has the most highly magnetic nucleus and because it makes up two thirds of the atoms in living tissues. It is largely the hydrogen in tissue water and body fat that is imaged by MRI.

Since its nucleus is the simplest, consisting of a single proton, imaging of hydrogen is often referred to as *proton imaging*. This can be misleading because all other nuclei, which are more complex, also contain protons; but in imaging terminology, they are identified by the chemical name of the

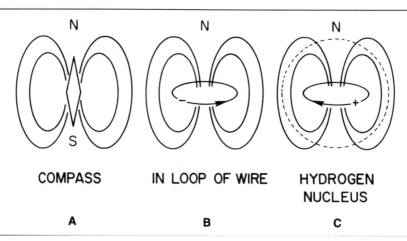

Figure 5A, B + C. (A) A compass needle is an example of a permanent magnet.
(B) Magnetic field produced by electric current in a loop of wire is an example of electromagnetism.
(C) In the hydrogen nucleus, movement of electric charge also creates magnetic field. The positive charge is located off-center, somewhere within the volume of the nucleus. Because the nucleus is spinning about an axis, the moving charge behaves like the current in the loop of wire, producing a magnetic field. This is nuclear magnetism.

atom, such as phosphorus or fluorine. In this book, "hydrogen nucleus" is used for "proton."

Why should the nuclei of some atoms be magnetic? A permanent magnet such as a compass needle or bar magnet produces a surrounding magnetic field (Figure 5A). Magnetic fields are always created by the movement of electrical charges, either positive or negative. This is true even in a permanent magnet, where the field is produced by orbiting electrons locked into the crystalline structure of the magnet.

When a current of electrons (negative charges) passes through a piece of straight wire, a magnetic field surrounds the wire. If we bend the wire into a circular loop, a magnetic field similar to that of a bar magnet is created (Figure 5B).

For our purposes, we may consider that the nucleus of the hydrogen atom is a very small volume of space containing a positive electrical charge. Due to two properties of the hydrogen nucleus, the electrical charge creates a magnetic field analogous to that produced by a loop of wire carrying moving charges. One of these properties is that the positive charge is located at some distance away from the center of the nucleus; the other is a property called *spin*.

The term spin, as used in classical physics, refers to the rotation of an object about an axis. When used in nuclear physics, spin describes a roughly analogous phenomenon. Spin is an inherent property of fundamental particles and, like nuclear mass, does not change.

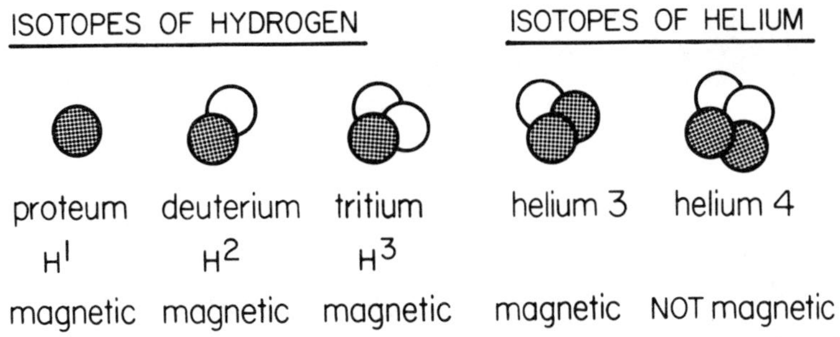

ISOTOPES OF HYDROGEN   ISOTOPES OF HELIUM

proteum   deuterium   tritium   helium 3   helium 4
H^1 H^2 H^3
magnetic   magnetic   magnetic   magnetic   NOT magnetic

Figure 6. A nucleus is some combination of protons and neutrons. When it contains either an unpaired proton or neutron, or both, it has net spin and is therefore magnetic.

The five simplest nuclei are shown, the protons black and the neutrons white. A pair of protons or a pair of neutrons have opposed spins which cancel each other (as in helium 4). To be magnetic, a nucleus must have an unpaired proton (as in all three isotopes of hydrogen) or an unpaired neutron (as in helium 3) or one of each (as in deuterium).

We can think of the hydrogen nucleus as physically spinning about an axis, but unlike familiar objects in the real world, its rate of rotation is unknown and it is not slowing down due to friction. Its positive charge is not located at the exact center of the nucleus but is located some distance from the axis, so that as the nucleus spins, the positive charge revolves in an approximately circular path, much as the electron in a loop of wire. This movement of the positive charge produces a magnetic field (Figure 5C).

Of the approximately 280 stable nuclei, about 100 are magnetic. The rule of thumb for determining whether or not a nucleus is magnetic is described in Figure 6.

The magnetism of these nuclei does not affect normal biochemical reactions. But under the conditions created in the MRI scanner, nuclear magnetism can be exploited for imaging.

The compass needle and hydrogen nucleus are very different, but they have enough in common to make comparison valid. When the hydrogen nucleus is placed in a strong magnetic field, it exhibits properties in many ways comparable to those of the compass needle in the Earth's magnetic field: It will tend to align with a magnetic field; it has a resonant frequency proportional to the external field strength; it absorbs energy (provided the energy is at the resonant frequency); and it will subsequently re-emit this energy.

In Chapter 1 we learned that a magnetic object (the compass needle) in a magnetic field exhibits magnetic resonance. When the resonating magnetic object is an atomic nucleus, this is nuclear magnetic resonance (NMR).

ALIGNMENT WITH EXTERNAL FIELD

The compass needle has a north and south pole and in the Earth's magnetic field aligns itself north-south. The hydrogen nucleus has a north and south

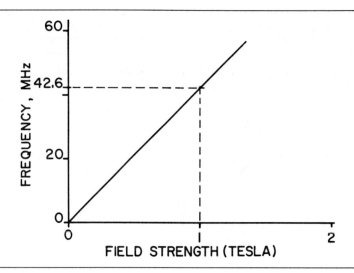

Figure 7. The resonant larmor frequency of the hydrogen nucleus is directly proportional to field strength.

pole and similarly tends to align itself with the MRI scanner's magnetic field.

RESONANT FREQUENCY

The frequency at which the hydrogen nucleus oscillates in a magnetic field is its resonant frequency, comparable to the frequency at which a compass needle oscillates in the Earth's magnetic field. A term commonly used for the resonant frequency of an atomic nucleus is *larmor frequency*, named after the British physicist Sir Joseph Larmor (1857–1942).

A compass needle in the earth's field might oscillate at one cycle per second. The resonant (larmor) frequency of the hydrogen nucleus in the magnetic field of the MRI scanner is many millions of times faster, due to the physical dimensions and magnetic properties of the hydrogen nucleus, and to the much stronger magnetic fields used. A typical high field-strength scanner might have a field strength of 10,000 gauss (one tesla). In this field, the resonant frequency of hydrogen is 42.6 million cycles per second (Figure 7).

STIMULATION

We were able to stimulate the compass needle into oscillation with a simple tap of our finger. The nucleus of a hydrogen atom is stimulated by another means: radio waves.

A radio wave is a weak magnetic field which reverses direction millions of times per second. This alternating magnetic field is created by a loop of wire in which the flow of current is reversed at the desired frequency. Each cycle of reversal is the equivalent of a single tap in the series of taps we used to stimulate a compass needle, or of a single push on a child's playground swing.

Radio waves travel at the speed of light and have a particular frequency (the number of cycles per second). For radio waves to be effective in stimulating hydrogen nuclei, the frequency of the radio waves must be tuned to the resonant frequency of the nuclei in a particular magnetic field strength. For the one tesla field mentioned above, the radio waves would need to be at 42.6 million cycles per second, a frequency located in the short wave radio band. The radio waves are applied to the hydrogen nuclei in short bursts or pulses lasting a small fraction of a second.

The absorption of energy from radio waves by a magnetic atomic nucleus constitutes the phenomenon of nuclear magnetic resonance.

DETECTION

The movement of the compass needle could be detected visually, but this is impossible in the case of the hydrogen nucleus. It is nonetheless possible to monitor its behavior: After stimulation by radio waves of the appropriate frequency, the hydrogen nucleus re-emits the absorbed energy, again in the form of radio waves. These re-emitted waves can be detected by a short-wave radio antenna and receiver.

Another way of explaining this emitted signal is that the nucleus, because it is an oscillating magnet, induces a voltage in an antenna. The signal from an individual nucleus is too weak to measure, but the signal from many millions of nuclei can be detected by the antenna of the MRI scanner. Quite remarkably, an MRI scanner uses only an ordinary short-wave radio transmitter and receiver to stimulate the tissue and detect the signal from which detailed pictures of the inside of the body are made.

The stimulation of the hydrogen nucleus and detection of its subsequent behavior can be likened to the percussion of a bell: A hammer is used to stimulate the bell, and the energy absorbed from the stimulation is subsequently emitted as sound. A further similarity between sound and NMR is the rate at which the energy is re-emitted. The rate at which the sound of a bell diminishes is comparable to the manner in which hydrogens in tissues re-emit radio energy. In living tissues, this energy falls off over a period of time lasting from perhaps a tenth of a second to a few seconds.

LOCALIZATION OF HYDROGEN NUCLEI

As with the compass needle, the resonant frequency of the stimulated hydrogen nucleus is proportional to the external field strength. In the case of the compass on the Earth's surface, the frequency of its swinging motion increased as we carried it up the magnetic gradient from the equator toward the north pole, where the magnetic field is stronger. With the hydrogen nucleus, the resonant frequency similarly increases with field strength. It is this relationship between the magnetic field strength and the resonant frequency of hydrogen nuclei which allows their localization.

Localization of hydrogen nuclei in the body is thus similar in principle to localization of a compass needle in the Earth's magnetic field: In a gradient magnetic field, the location of the hydrogen nucleus can be deduced from its resonant frequency. The Earth's field forms a natural gradient, but the magnetic field gradient required to image hydrogen nuclei is produced artificially by the MRI scanner.

Without these gradients, the entire anatomical region under examination would respond as a single entity and no localization within it would be possible. The way in which gradient magnetic fields are used to make clinically useful images is the subject of the next chapter.

CHAPTER 3: IMAGING

In the first figure of the introduction, we described the X-ray CT scan as accomplishing the following imaginary sequence of events: The head is frozen and a fine saw makes two transverse cuts one centimeter apart, thereby creating a cross-sectional slab of head one centimeter thick. This slice is removed intact, placed on high-contrast X-ray film, and exposed to a broad beam of X-rays at right angles to the slice of tissue. When the radiograph of the slice has been processed and placed on a viewbox, the image would be essentially the same as that produced by the CT scanner. The CT scanner produces these results without physically altering the head. Except for slight tissue ionization, this process is entirely harmless (Figure 1).

The MRI scan can be described in a similar imaginary fashion. After the frozen slice of tissue is removed, rather than a radiograph being made of it, it is physically cut up into tiny square cylinders called volume elements or voxels. Each is one millimeter on an edge and occupies a known position in the original slice of tissue (Figure 8). Each of these small square cylinders is (in effect) placed in a test tube which is then placed in a laboratory NMR apparatus, and its hydrogen nuclei analyzed. This imaginary exercise suggests the great analytic capability of the MRI process.

In this chapter, we discuss how MRI localizes these square cylinders of tissue and recombines them to make an image of the cross-sectional slice.

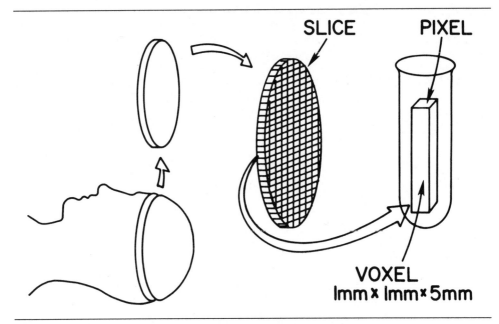

Figure 8. The MRI scan may be thought of as being produced by these steps: Freezing the body, cutting out a slab of tissue, slicing it up into small square cylindrical voxels, and placing each voxel in a test tube. The analysis of individual voxels symbolizes the considerable characterization possible by MRI.

PROPERTIES OF THE HYDROGEN NUCLEUS

In the previous chapter, we noted the properties of the hydrogen nucleus that are important to MRI:

1. In the presence of the strong magnetic field created in the MRI scanner, the hydrogen nuclei tend to align themselves with the field.
2. The hydrogen nuclei resonate at a frequency (the larmor frequency) which is proportional to the strength of the magnetic field.
3. In a gradient magnetic field (one that changes the strength of the main field between one position and another), the resonant frequency of the hydrogen nuclei indicates their location in the gradient.

The MRI scanner creates the strong fields necessary to align the hydrogen nuclei and the gradient fields necessary to localize them. The scanner has a radio transmitter to provide the stimulation (the pulse of radio waves) and an antenna to detect the radio waves re-emitted from the hydrogen nuclei following stimulation.

NMR IN A HOMOGENEOUS FIELD

We have emphasized the importance of gradient fields in MRI, but before proceeding to show how gradient fields are used to create an image of a

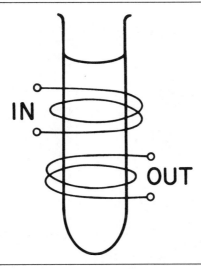

Figure 9. To demonstrate the phenomenon of NMR requires only a simple apparatus. A small test tube filled with a homogeneous sample (water) is placed in a uniform one tesla field, and two loops of wire are wrapped around it. One acts as a radio transmitter, exposing the sample to radio energy at the resonant frequency of the hydrogen, and the other as a radio antenna, which measures the radio signal reradiated from the sample. Because the test tube is exposed to a uniform magnetic field, the entire sample responds similarly.

cross-sectional slice, it might be helpful to examine the behavior of a homogeneous sample of hydrogen nuclei in a uniform field. To do this, we could use a simple apparatus similar to that used by Felix Bloch and Robert Purcell, who independently described the phenomenon of NMR in 1946.

In this device, a small sample of a homogeneous substance — in this case water in test tube — is placed in the apparatus. The magnetic field applied to the sample is designed to be the same strength throughout the sample. Each hydrogen nucleus in the test tube experiences the same one tesla field and consequently has the same resonant frequency (42.6 million cycles per second) regardless of its location. When a stimulating pulse of 42.6 million cycle per second radio waves is applied to the sample, the entire sample absorbs the radio-frequency energy. Subsequently, the entire sample re-emits energy. Because the magnetic field is held constant, the hydrogen nuclei re-emit the energy as 42.6 million cycle per second radio waves (Figure 9).

An analysis of this re-emitted signal provides information about the hydrogen nuclei: The strength of the signal indicates concentration; the observed rate of fading of the signal also tells much about impurities in the water (this will be covered in more detail in the next chapter). However, because all of the hydrogen nuclei in the sample respond identically, the signal contains no information that would help localize hydrogen within the sample (Figure 10).

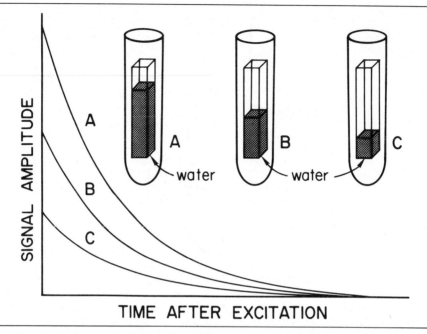

Figure 10. Voxels containing 75%, 50%, and 25% water (respectively) are excited by a radio pulse at the hydrogen resonant frequency. The signal returned from each sample is proportional to the amount of water in the test tube. Measuring regional hydrogen distribution is the simplest MRI analysis.

IMAGING A CROSS SECTION OF TISSUE

The following shows how, in a gradient magnetic field, the properties of hydrogen nuclei are used to image a transverse slice of tissue. (Although a transverse slice is used as an example, imaging of planes in any orientation is possible.) What follows is a description of the most common method of MRI excitation and data manipulation. Many modifications of this basic method have been described, but the principles are much the same.

The first step in imaging a transverse slice is isolation of that slice from other tissues. This corresponds to the first step in the imaginary analogy described above: the sawing of the slice of tissue from the body. The most common method of imaging uses gradients to selectively excite an individual slice. After its excitation, further information is obtained by creating new gradients within the slice itself.

Isolation of a Transverse Slice of Tissue

To isolate this slice, the scanner creates a magnetic gradient longitudinally through the body, from head to foot, along what is usually termed the Z-axis. We will arbitrarily say that the field is stronger toward the head and weaker toward the feet. In practice, the magnetic gradients used in MRI are weak, changing strength by about one gauss per centimeter, which in a one

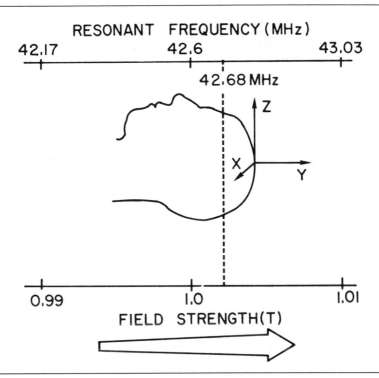

Figure 11. The head is placed in a longitudinal gradient, which is weaker on the left and stronger on the right. The resonant frequencies of hydrogen nuclei vary according to their position in the gradient; a single resonant frequency corresponds to a single transverse plane. When the entire head is exposed to a radio signal of 42.68 megahertz, only the hydrogens in a single transverse slice of tissue (dashed line) are stimulated.

tesla field is a change of only 0.01% per centimeter. The resonance of the hydrogen nucleus is so sharply defined that even such a slight change in field strength is all that is needed to isolate a plane a few millimeters thick. It is impractical to create a sufficiently controlled gradient through the entire body, so the gradient is generated only in the region being imaged.

In the presence of this gradient, the hydrogens in the body become spatially encoded, i.e., there is a relationship between their resonant frequency and their position in the gradient. In this example, the hydrogen nuclei in each successively rostral (toward the head) transverse plane of the body are exposed to progressively higher field strengths, and so resonate at correspondingly higher larmor frequencies. In this example, there is only one plane of tissue exposed to exactly one tesla field strength (Figure 11).

If the entire anatomical region is exposed to a radio signal of 42.6 million cycles per second, only those hydrogen nuclei lying within the one tesla plane of tissue will absorb the energy of the radio waves and be stimulated. Hydrogen nuclei in adjacent slices of tissue remain unstimulated and silent. If we wished to isolate a slice of tissue higher or lower in the body, we would adjust the frequency of the radio signal to a higher or lower frequency, accordingly. We could also move the slice by changing the gradient in relation to the body.

In this way, through the application of a gradient to the body and the exposure of the tissue to a radio signal of a single frequency, the hydrogen nuclei in only a single transverse slice are stimulated. The plane is thus isolated from neighboring, unstimulated tissue.

If the Z-axis is longitudinal through the body, any transverse plane can be described, using the cartesian coordinate system: The excited slice of tissue lies in the X-Y plane.

In this theoretical discussion, we have used a stimulating pulse of radio signal containing only a single frequency. This would produce an infinitesimally thin slice of tissue and thus an unusably weak re-emitted signal. In practice, the stimulating pulse would also contain radio frequencies slightly above and below the frequency at the center of the slice. This increases the thickness of the imaged section and increases its signal output.

Localization within the Transverse Slice

At this point we have isolated a slice of tissue by stimulating the hydrogens in one plane of the body. As noted, the hydrogen nuclei start to re-emit the signal immediately after stimulation. However, simply stopping the imaging process at this point and listening to the signal would not provide useful imaging data. The intensity of the signal would simply indicate the average signal from all regions of the slice.

To further localize the nuclei within the excited slice, new gradients (in different directions) are used.

After the transverse slice of tissue has been isolated and the hydrogens in it stimulated, the head-to-toe Z-axis gradient and the radio-frequency excitation are turned off. The re-radiated signal appears. A second gradient is then created, this time transversely across the body (at right angles to the Z-axis) in the X-Y plane. As a result, the field on one edge of the slice being imaged is stronger than on the other. How the scanner creates this second gradient will be discussed in Chapter 6. Here, it is important to know only that the transverse gradient can be in any direction across the isolated slice. For simplicity, in the figure it is shown increasing from left to right along the X-axis, shoulder to shoulder (Figure 12).

The result of applying a transverse gradient is that the nuclei in the isolated slice of tissue, which had all been oscillating at the same frequency, now find themselves in magnetic fields of differing strengths. The nuclei resonate at new frequencies (higher or lower) depending on their position in the transverse gradient at that instant of time. Again the resonant frequencies of the nuclei are spatially encoded so that nuclei at one edge of the slice, in the weaker end of the gradient field, resonate at lower frequencies than those at

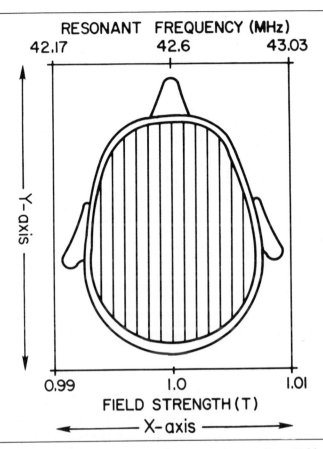

Figure 12. The isolated plane of tissue is exposed to a transverse gradient. Field strength along the X-axis gradient is shown at bottom, and the corresponding hydrogen frequencies at the top. Nuclei along one line have the same resonant frequency.

the other edge, in the stronger field. Thus the excited transverse section of tissue is sliced into parallel strips, the nuclei along any one strip resonating at the same frequency.

A comparable spatial encoding of position by frequency is found in the ordinary piano, in which keys on the left correspond to lower notes and keys on the right to higher (Figure 13). The location of the string on the piano can be determined from the frequency (pitch) of the note produced by the vibrating string.

The second magnetic gradient is applied immediately after the original Z-axis gradient is turned off, while the hydrogens are still "ringing" from their initial stimulation. When they take up their new resonant frequencies in the second gradient, they continue to emit radio-frequency signals without further stimulation. The frequencies of the signals emitted, however, correspond to those of the new field strength of the gradient at each location, each frequency representing a line across the slice.

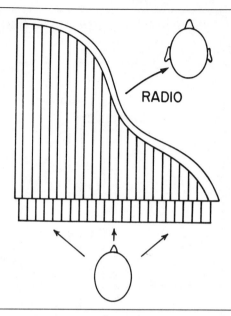

Figure 13. A piano is an example of spatial encoding by frequency. To the left of the keyboard the notes are lower, to the right, higher. Even over the radio, we can determine the location of the strings from their pitch.

Regardless of the initial frequency of stimulation, subsequent frequency of oscillation of the nucleus changes with the field strength. In this way it is like a guitar string being tuned, whose pitch instantaneously changes with changing tension on the string (Figure 14).

The radio signal emitted from the plane now contains a mix of frequencies. By measuring the strength of the radio signal at the different frequencies, the amount of hydrogen along each line in the slice of tissue can be determined.

This plane of tissue divided into parallel lines, each line of tissue radiating a specific frequency of radio waves at a particular intensity, can again be compared to a piano. In this case, all of the strings of the piano are vibrating, each producing its own note. Such a mix of notes would be a meaningless jumble, even to a skilled musician. With the help of electronic frequency analyzers, however, this cacophony could be analyzed into intelligible information. The individual notes could be distinguished and their respective volumes measured. We would know which notes were being played and at what volume. From this we would know the location of the strings and how hard the corresponding keys had been struck (Figure 15).

In MRI such electronic frequency analyzers are used to analyze the radio signal radiating from the tissue. This analysis determines which frequencies are being radiated from the tissues and at what intensities. The frequency tells us the location of the line and the amplitude of the total number of hydrogen nuclei along that line.

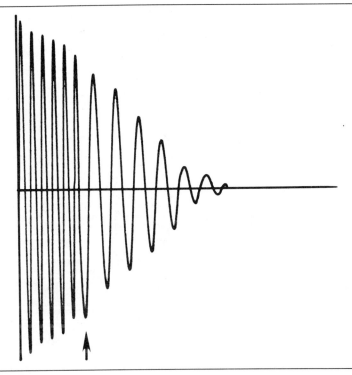

Figure 14. The sound from a guitar string being tuned. The guitar string is plucked, and initially oscillates (vibrates) at a specific frequency. The tension on the string is subsequently lowered (small vertical arrow). Its frequency of oscillation slows; the pitch of the note drops.

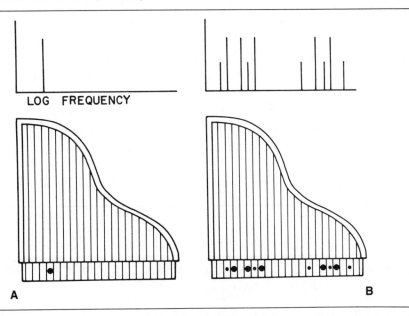

LOG FREQUENCY

A

B

Figure 15A + B. (A) Electronic analysis of the sound from a piano on which a single key has been struck (indicated by the black dot on the keyboard). A single peak shows on the electronic display.
(B) Frequency analysis of the sound from a piano on which many keys have been struck with differing intensities (indicated by size of black dot on keyboard). Electronic analysis shows a peak for each key struck. Height of peak indicates how hard the key was struck.

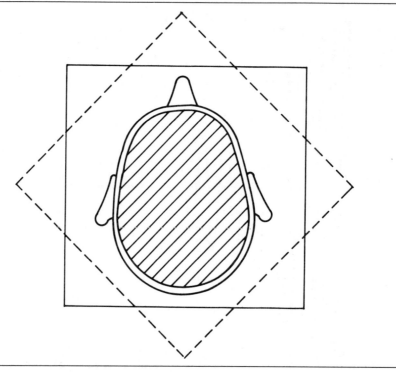

Figure 16. In order to gather enough data to form an image, a single slice of tissue must be examined many times, each time using a transverse gradient oriented in a different direction. Each change of direction defines the number of hydrogens along a new set of parallel lines. Two gradient directions are indicated here by the solid and dashed lines.

Rotation of Transverse Gradient

After the data from one pulse have all been recovered and stored in the computer, the process described above is repeated, starting with the restoration of the Z-axis gradient.

The same transverse slice of tissue across the head is again excited by radio frequency energy. After the stimulating pulse, the Z-axis gradient is again turned off, and the transverse gradient is applied across the isolated slice of tissue, but this time in a slightly different direction. In this way the hydrogen concentration along a new set of parallel strips, slightly askew to the first set, is measured (Figure 16).

In the course of scanning one slice of tissue, this process is repeated many times; each time the transverse gradient is applied to the slice of tissue at a slightly different angle, so that by the end of the scan, the slice of tissue has been cut into a few hundred sets of parallel lines, each set crossing the plane of the slice at a different angle.

Computer Reconstruction

At this point, we have isolated the slice of tissue from the body and cut it into parallel strips, but we have yet to divide each strip into individual

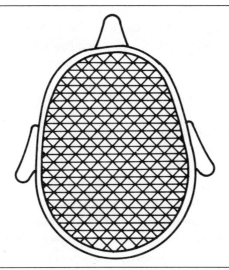

Figure 17. During the course of this type of MRI scan, the transverse gradient is rotated many times by a few degrees at a time. The image is reconstructed from the thousands of intersecting lines.

volumes of tissue (voxels) and measure their hydrogen concentration, as we had proposed. This last step in the imaging process is accomplished by the computer.

When the instrumentation in the MRI scanner measures the total amount of hydrogen along a particular strip of tissue in the slice being imaged, the measurement is stored in the computer. Graphically, we can think of this strip as a line having a shade of gray or *brightness* that depends on the total amount of hydrogen in the corresponding strip of tissue. During the imaging of one slice of tissue, thousands of such lines of varying brightness are stored in the computer. Any one voxel in the tissue slice represents the intersection of hundreds of lines (Figure 17).

One might think that the simple superimposition of these lines would result in a useable picture. It would be reasonable to assume that if any one voxel in the plane is high in hydrogen concentration, then all the lines passing through it would be correspondingly bright. Superimposing these lines should (intuitively) produce a correspondingly bright pixel and, perhaps, a useable picture, but this is not the case. In fact, such simple superimposition, without further manipulation by computation, results in a blurred and useless picture.

To produce a useable picture, the computer carries out a classical mathematical maneuver — the Fourier transform — to reconstruct a clinically useful picture from the data. This involves essentially the same set of instructions (algorithm) used in reconstructing a CT image. The details of the Fourier transform and its applications to computer reconstruction of medical images is beyond the scope of this work (see Oldendorf 1980).

COMPARISON OF MRI AND CT COMPUTER RECONSTRUCTION

It is important to point out that the similarities between the computer reconstruction in CT and MRI arise from similarities in the data: Both techniques measure some average characteristic along a large number of intersecting lines.

Both modalities provide a means for isolating a slice of tissue from the body. In CT, the slice of tissue is isolated by a narrow beam of X-rays, the thickness of the slice of tissue being determined by the width of the X-ray beam. In MRI, the slice of tissue is isolated by radio waves used in combination with a magnetic gradient; hydrogen nuclei in only one slice of tissue respond to stimulation. The thickness of the slice is determined by the range of frequencies used in the exciting radio signal.

CT measures the total density of tissues in a narrow column of tissue interposed between the X-ray source and detector. In the older (first generation) models of the rotate-translate CT scanner, the X-ray source and detector were located on opposite sides of the head and their movement locked together, thereby making measurements along many columns of tissue lying parallel to each other in the plane of the tissue slice.

After making one translation movement across the head, the orientation of the X-ray source and detector was changed, so that the next set of measurements was of a new set of parallel columns of tissues, slightly askew to the previous set. The measurements were all stored in the computer and, as in MRI, represented graphically as a set of parallel lines of varying shades of gray. Each line had a position, direction, and a brightness representing the total number of X-ray deletions along the corresponding line through the patient, but giving no information about the desired structural detail.

In a similar fashion, in MRI the direction of the transverse magnetic gradient applied across the slice of tissue can be changed in a step-wise fashion, a few degrees each time, to produce many intersecting lines, representing the number of hydrogen nuclei along many paths through the plane under examination.

Again, the exact location of each hydrogen cannot be determined, but their total along each line is measured. The same computerized reconstruction as in X-ray CT is then applied, with the production of a two-dimensional MRI image which superficially resembles a CT scan. In this case, however, the images represent the distribution of hydrogen. As will be seen in Chapter 4, the data-gathering strategy may be modified to display other tissue characteristics (Figure 18).

In the case of CT, changes in direction of successive sweeps through tissue can be made only by physically moving the X-ray source. This greatly complicates design, construction, and maintenance and confines CT to imaging in the transverse plane. The change in direction of the magnetic field gradients in MRI scanning, however, does not require any physical movement, because it can be accomplished electronically using no moving parts.

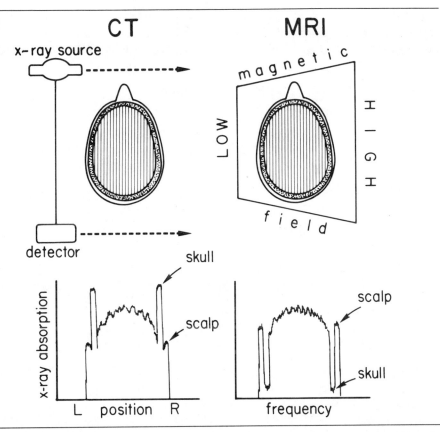

Figure 18. Because CT and MRI both take measurements along many lines crossing a plane of tissue, both use essentially the same computer algorithm to reconstruct an image. MRI measures the number of hydrogen nuclei along each line of tissue; CT measures X-ray absorption between source and detector.

One major difference between CT and MRI is shown by the lower profiles: Whereas bone in skull strongly absorbs X-rays (and appears bright on CT scans), no radio signal is emitted by bone in MRI (so skull is comparatively black).

One result of this is that MRI is not confined like CT to transverse slices, but can also image coronal or sagittal slices (as well as any other orientation), since the gradients can be used to create any examination plane desired. Although in this chapter the imaging of a transverse slice of tissue was used as an example, in MRI it is no more difficult to image other planes. For example, instead of the first gradient being applied longitudinally along the body, it can be applied transversely across the body to produce a sagittal section or front-to-back for a coronal section.

The use of linear gradients to localize the source of an NMR signal in a plane was described by Lauterbur (1973), and this opened the door to a variety of embellishments of his fundamental approach. The material in this chapter describes essentially Lauterbur's original work and is intended to introduce the principles of MRI.

In this example a single excitation pulse was used, and the amplitude of the signal measured, to produce an image of hydrogen distribution. A single pulse is rarely used in modern imaging; as described in Chapter 4, two or more pulses are usually used to emphasize other characteristics of the hydrogen nucleus and so better characterize tissues.

CHAPTER 4: TISSUE CHARACTERIZATION: T_1 AND T_2

Up to this point, we have discussed only one aspect of human MRI — the mapping of hydrogen concentration. If this were the only capability of MRI, it might not be worth the major effort already undertaken to develop clinical scanners. The great potential of MRI derives from its ability to provide several means of characterizing normal and pathological tissues.

We ordinarily think of tissue analysis as the measurement of the amount of a given substance per unit volume of tissue, for example, the amount of glucose in a volume of serum. CT measures regional specific gravity and iodine concentration.

Since in MRI the signal strength after a single pulse is proportional to the number of hydrogen nuclei, the simplest method of scanning shows distribution of hydrogen nuclei. Most hydrogens are in tissue water and fat. In practice, such simple hydrogen content turns out to be of little interest, because there is much hydrogen in essentially all tissues and little regional contrast is seen.

The useful information lies almost entirely in the *behavior* of regional hydrogen, rather than in its regional concentration. What is meant here by behavior is: how the hydrogen nucleus responds to influences from its chemical environment. The chemical environment changes the behavior of the hydrogen nucleus, which in turn changes qualities of the radio signal emitted by the tissues.

The idea of using the hydrogen nucleus to tell us about its environment could be clarified by a simple analogy. Through experience, we have learned how people respond to changes in the weather. Imagine that you awaken in a hotel room in a strange city and wish to know what the weather is like outside. If you looked out the window and could see people on the street below, you could infer much about the weather by observing their behavior. They serve as a behavioral probe of the weather. How are they dressed? If they are without coats it is probably warm. If they have umbrellas opened, it is most likely raining. If they are rushing about, it has probably just begun to rain. If they seek shelter in protected areas, it probably is windy. There are many other inferences about the weather that could be drawn from human behavior. Simply counting the people would be only a crude indicator of the weather.

In MRI we are observing the hydrogen nucleus and inferring characteristics of its magnetic environment from its behavior (in response to standardized radio-frequency stimulation). By varying the nature of our probing we can elicit different types of information. The behavior of hydrogen nuclei becomes a surprisingly rich source of information about the magnetic "weather" in the tissues.

CHANGES IN BEHAVIOR DUE TO LOCAL MAGNETIC FIELDS

To show how the behavior of hydrogen nuclei allows us to infer their environment, we might return briefly to the compass analogy. (We must first emphasize that the compass is only a crude approximation of the properties of the hydrogen nucleus. A large number of compass needles behave collectively like a large number of hydrogen nuclei; but while a single compass needle is used to make a point, it is not closely representative of the processes involved with a single hydrogen nucleus.)

At different parallels of latitude, the compass needle swings or oscillates at different resonant frequencies, because field strength varies with distance from the poles. If we carry the compass needle to different locations along the same latitude, we would expect it to oscillate at exactly the same frequency, since any point at that latitude is equally distant from the pole and should experience the same strength magnetic field.

In fact, we would find that the resonant frequency of the compass varies slightly with even minor changes of location. These changes are due to small local variations in the strength of the Earth's field. At one location, the compass might be near a natural deposit of iron ore, at another it might be inside a building with steel beams. These factors would change the strength of the magnetic field experienced by the compass needle.

RELAXATION TIMES

The hydrogen nucleus exposed to the magnetic field created by the MRI scanner likewise experiences small local variations in magnetic field strength. These fluctuations occur on a submolecular level, due to the presence of magnetic nuclei and atoms. Hydrogen nuclei are themselves weakly magnetic, but there are also some entire atoms in tissues, such as manganese and dissolved oxygen, which are very strongly magnetic. The nuclear magnetism of water hydrogen and other atoms is not obvious, since it is not apparent in ordinary physiology, but these magnetic objects significantly alter the magnetic microenvironment of the water hydrogens being imaged. These effects are the weather in our earlier hotel window analogy. It is the ability to detect these differences in the magnetic environment of the hydrogen nucleus that gives MRI its great diagnostic potential.

These alterations in behavior modify the signal received after excitation. There are two observable aspects of behavior of the hydrogen nucleus that are affected by the local magnetic environment: These are termed *time constants* T_1 and T_2, which are also referred to as *relaxation times*, because they define the rate at which the emitted signal fades after stimulation. T_1 and T_2 represent two largely independent processes, each of which contributes to fading of the signal following excitation.

TIME CONSTANT T_1 (COMPASS NEEDLE)

To understand T_1, we can examine the behavior of one compass needle on the Earth's surface. We stimulate the compass needle by tapping it with our finger. At first it swings in a wide arc as it oscillates. Over a period of several seconds, the needle loses energy to bearing friction and air drag, swinging in progressively shorter arcs until it finally comes to rest pointing north. The compass needle, being a small magnet, induces a faint but detectable signal in an antenna coil placed near it. The signal diminishes as the swinging motion diminishes. For mathematical reasons, we define T_1 as the time it takes for the induced signal to fall by 63% from its original strength (Figure 19).

TIME CONSTANT T_2 (COMPASS NEEDLE)

Imagine that we have several identical compasses, located at different points on the same parallel of latitude on the Earth's surface. We stimulate them simultaneously so that they swing in unison. We would expect the motion of all the compass needles to decay at the same rate, and their combined signal to fall off at the same rate as that produced by a single compass, but this is not the case.

The combined signal falls off much faster than expected, due to the phenomenon of dephasing. Although the compass needles would all initially be swinging together (in phase), unavoidable local variations in magnetic field strength cause them to swing at slightly different rates; after a few seconds they are no longer in phase. Even though each compass is still swinging, the signal produced by any one compass needle partially cancels that produced by another. Consequently, over a period of a few seconds, the combined signal falls off more quickly than the signal from a single compass. T_2 is defined as the time it takes for dephasing to weaken the signal by 63%.

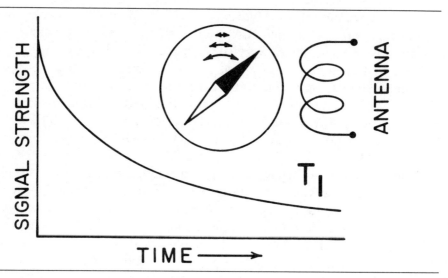

Figure 19. The swinging compass needle loses energy due to friction and air drag, eventually returning to rest in its original position in the Earth's field. An external antenna measures T_1, the rate of decay.

We should note that the measured signal can disappear due to dephasing, even though individually the compasses have not lost their energy (Figure 20).

It is easy to find examples of mutual reinforcement of multiple weak signals. A platoon of soldiers might be walking along a road some distance from an observer. The sound of their boots on the road might not be audible if they were simply walking out of step with each other. If, however, they were marching in step, the clumping sound of their individual boots would reinforce each other and they could then be audible at this distance. To say they are marching in step is a way of stating they are marching in phase, or that they are phase coherent.

LOSS OF ENERGY

T_1 measures the rate of loss of energy; it is important to note that the compass actually loses energy as the oscillation decays and the needle comes back to rest pointing north. In T_2, there is no energy loss; the weakening of the emitted signal occurs as a group effect, the result of dephasing (a loss of coherence) between the compasses. They are still swinging individually, but the combined signal falls off.

Hydrogen nuclei, in the aggregate, also exhibit these two properties. The decay of the observed signal occurs due to the combined effects of T_1 and T_2. Fortunately, it is possible to measure the contributions of T_1 and T_2 independently.

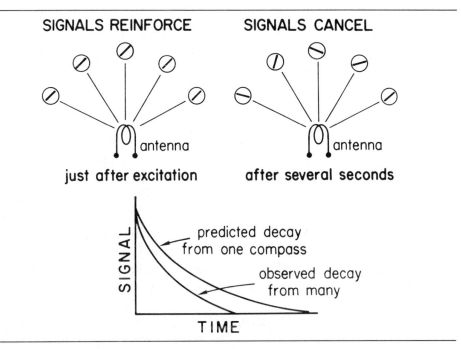

Figure 20. Initially a group of compass needles swing in phase with each other, but local variations in magnetic field strength cause them to oscillate at slightly differing rates. As they drift out of phase, their combined signal falls off at rate T_2.

T_1 AND T_2 IN MRI

To some extent it is possible to isolate a compass needle from extraneous magnetic influences so that it responds only to the Earth's magnetic field. It is impossible to isolate a hydrogen molecule (and its nucleus) from local magnetic influences so that it responds only to the field of the MRI scanner. In the watery environment of the tissues, water molecules are in constantly changing contact with other magnetic nuclei and atoms. Such magnetic atoms can have a strong influence on the magnetic properties of the hydrogen nuclei. The most we can do to reduce extraneous magnetic influences is to remove magnetic impurities from the water, but even in pure water, the magnetic hydrogen nuclei influence each other.

When the human body is exposed to the brief stimulating pulse from the MRI scanner's radio transmitter, many trillions of nuclei are stimulated in the slice of tissue being imaged. Immediately, two processes start: the re-emission of energy measured as T_1 and the dephasing of hydrogen nuclei measured as T_2. The radio signal re-emitted from the tissues is measured by the MRI scanner's antenna and radio receiver. The complex microenvironments of living tissues have a strong influence on the magnetic properties of water molecules: Both T_1 and T_2 are greatly shortened, relative to pure water, and the signal falls off correspondingly faster.

T_1 of Hydrogen

T_1 is defined as the time it takes for the hydrogen nuclei to emit 63% of the energy they absorbed from a stimulating pulse. At field strengths ordinarily used in MRI scanners, the T_1 of pure water is about 2.5–3 seconds.

T_2 of Hydrogen

One effect of the stimulating radio frequency pulse is to make all of the hydrogen nuclei oscillate more or less in phase with each other, just as tapping a group of compass needles simultaneously made them swing synchronously. Immediately after the excitation, they are maximally in phase. As they continue to oscillate, movement of magnetic nuclei and atoms creates minute, fluctuating local magnetic fields. These cause the nuclei to oscillate at slightly differing frequencies, and they drift out of phase. Eventually they become completely out of phase with each other.

When the individual nuclei oscillate out of phase, the radio waves they emit are also out of phase and so cancel each other. As a result, the signal detected by the MRI scanner, the sum of radio signals from trillions of nuclei, falls off more quickly than if the nuclei were unaffected by local fluctuations. T_2 is defined as the time for 63% of the signal to be lost due to dephasing. T_2 of pure water is also about 2.5–3 seconds. T_2 must always be shorter than or equal to T_1, since phase relationship is of no interest once the nuclei have all lost their energy.

FACTORS AFFECTING T_1 AND T_2

The local fluctuations in magnetic field strength that alter magnetic behavior of hydrogen nuclei come from thermal motion of magnetic particles.

Thermal Motion

The environment of the nucleus is a world of violent motion. At body temperature, water and other molecules that make up the magnetic environment are in constant motion, colliding randomly with each other.

The most obvious aspect of this thermal motion is Brownian motion, which was first observed by Scottish botanist Robert Brown in 1827 while examining a suspension of pollen grains under a microscope. A pollen grain or other small particle undergoes visible random movement as though buffeted by invisible particles. In the vicinity of the particle are many very much smaller water molecules, bombarding its surface millions of times per second. These impacts on the particle largely cancel each other, but since they are random in time they sometimes impact unequally on two sides of the particle. The result is a jiggling motion of the particle which is low enough in frequency and has enough displacement to be visible with any good microscope. Anyone interested in MRI should seek out an ordinary laboratory microscope and observe India ink (diluted 1:100) at 400–1000

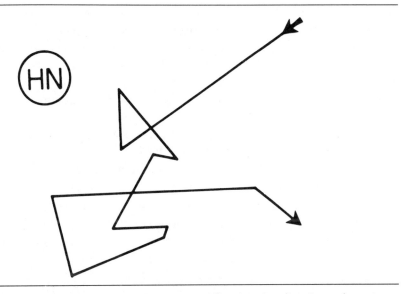

Figure 21. In the liquid state a water molecule moves rapidly, changing direction and rotating as it undergoes many collisions and near-collisions.

magnification. The vigorous motion of the carbon particles that make the ink black is very impressive. It is a direct observation of thermal motion, the basis of both T_1 and T_2 relaxation.

Water molecules undergo similar random collisions with each other but at a much faster rate (Figure 21). It is important to note that in addition to direct collisions, many near-collisions occur.

Since water molecules contain two magnetic hydrogen nuclei, each interaction of one water molecule with another — whether a collision or near-collison — is a magnetic event, resulting in a brief fluctuation of the magnetic field experienced by each nucleus. Because a water molecule undergoes many millions of collisions per second, each nucleus experiences many millions of magnetic fluctuations. The hydrogen nuclei in the tissues respond to this magnetic signal, as they did to the electromagnetic radio waves from the MRI scanner's radio transmitter during stimulation.

Whereas the signal produced by a radio transmitter is well controlled, consisting of cycles of fluctuation of the same intensity at evenly-spaced intervals, the nature of the magnetic signal produced by thermal motion is much more complex. The collisions or near-misses between water molecules occur randomly, so the fluctuations in the magnetic signal are random. How close the water molecules come to each other in near-collisions is also variable, so the intensity of the fluctuations is correspondingly variable. In addition, other aspects of the molecule's motion create magnetic perturbations. First, each collision changes the speed, as well as the direction, of the water molecule. Second, the molecule undergoes a rotational tumbling motion as it moves. These additional motions of the water molecules further complicate the magnetic fluctuations, or signal, experienced by other water molecules.

Consequently, the magnetic field produced within a region of water by thermal motion is extremely complex. It can be thought of as a mixture of magnetic fluctuations covering a wide range of frequencies.

The complexity of these randomly-produced magnetic influences can be compared to the familiar phenomenon of audible white noise. When an inflated tire is punctured, we hear a hiss as the air escapes into the atmosphere. The hissing is the result of the turbulence created when the rapid stream of air emerges from the hole and is broken into many vortices. This turbulence is a random phenomenon which produces a wide range of audible frequencies, called white noise. The term *white noise* is borrowed from the field of optics, which tells us that the color white is produced by a mixture of all frequencies (colors) of visible light.

In tissues, the complex thermal motion of water molecules produces a comparable phenomenon, a magnetic signal containing fluctuations occurring at many frequencies. This is the environment of magnetic white noise to which the hydrogen nucleus responds during the MRI imaging process.

The responses of hydrogen nuclei to environmental magnetic fluctuations determine the rate of energy loss (T_1) and the rate of dephasing (T_2) during MRI.

Effect of thermal motion on T_2

Because the effect of thermal motion on the T_2 of hydrogen is more easily explained than for T_1, it is presented here first.

We have studied how the resonant larmor frequency of the hydrogen nucleus depends on the strength of the magnetic field it experiences. In MRI scanning, almost all of this field is produced by the scanner itself. However, thermal motion of the tissue water is constantly creating minute fluctuations superimposed on this main field. Any fluctuation results in a corresponding change in the resonant frequency and causes the nucleus to oscillate slightly faster or slower. Since no two nuclei experience the same fluctuations, the oscillations of the nuclei, over a period of time, drift out of phase with each other (Figure 22).

During MRI imaging, large populations of hydrogen nuclei are stimulated by a pulse of radio-frequency energy and subsequently re-emit the energy, again as radio waves. The received signal is not representative of this re-emission, because the nuclear sources of the signal go rapidly out of phase and the emitted energy seems to disappear long before it actually does.

To summarize the loss of signal due to dephasing: Immediately after stimulation the larmor precessions of the nuclei are most in phase. At this time, the emitted radio waves (which, when summed, create the observed signal) are in phase, and the signal is strongest. Because the nuclei drift out

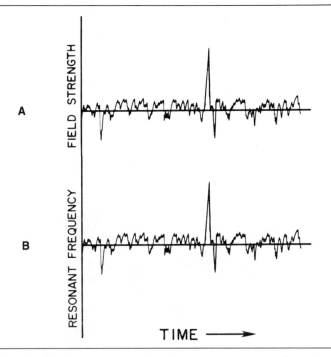

Figure 22A + B. (A) Random fluctuations in field strength at a particular nucleus due to the thermal motion of magnetic nuclei and atoms. In this imaginary graph, the large spike represents a near miss with a strongly magnetic atom.
(B) The resonant frequency of the nucleus varies, precisely following changes in field strength. The random change in resonant frequency of each nucleus causes the degradation of phase relationship between nuclei, thereby determining T_2.

of phase due to thermal motion, the emitted radio waves drift out of phase and cancel each other, so the radio signal falls off quickly. When they are completely out of phase (randomly phased), no signal is received. The rate of dephasing is defined by T_2, the time it takes for the dephasing to cause the signal to fall by 63%.

It is important to note that T_2 is shortened by magnetic noise fluctuations of *any* frequency.

Effect of thermal motion on T_1

Hydrogen nuclei being imaged by MRI are stimulated by radio waves tuned to the resonant frequency of the nuclei. (In a one tesla field, the resonant larmor frequency of hydrogen nuclei is 42.6 million cycles per second.)

Some very small component of the magnetic white noise caused by thermal motion occurs at the larmor frequency at which the hydrogen nucleus is oscillating. We might expect that magnetic fluctuations at the resonant frequency of the nuclei would evoke a special response from the energized nuclei. This is indeed the case. For reasons explained in the Appendix, magnetic fluctuations at this particular frequency cause the population of

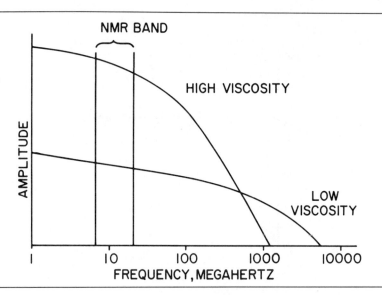

Figure 23. The two curves represent the frequency distribution of the magnetic fluctuations due to thermal motion. At low viscosity (or high temperature), the thermal motion is faster; there are more high frequency components. The area under the two curves is the same.

The hydrogen resonant frequency falls somewhere in the NMR band, depending on the strength of the magnet in the scanner. At high viscosity (or lower temperature), thermal motion slows; more of the fluctuations occur in the NMR band.

stimulated hydrogen nuclei to lose their energy faster than in the absence of these fluctuations. The magnetic signal triggers the release of energy. This type of event is known as a *stimulated emission*.

While T_2 is affected by magnetic noise fluctuations at *any* frequency, T_1 is affected *only* by those at the resonant larmor frequency.

Thermal motion and temperature

Thermal motion produces (for pure water) a range of frequencies starting at zero and extending up into the thousands of millions of cycles per second, far above any larmor frequencies likely to be found in imaging.
water) a range of frequencies starting at zero and extending up into the thousands of millions of cycles per second, far above any larmor frequencies likely to be found in imaging.

In commercial MRI scanners, the resonant larmor frequency falls somewhere in the range of 1–85 million cycles per second, the specific frequency being determined by the strength of the main magnet.

Only a small fraction of the magnetic field thermal fluctuations occurs at the lower larmor frequencies likely to be used in MRI, and a very small fraction of this occurs at the specific larmor frequency of any one scanner. This small component at the larmor frequency does, however, trigger the hydrogens being imaged by MRI to lose their energy. The strength of this particular frequency component thus determines T_1.

The thermal motion of pure water at body temperature tends to be "high-pitched," most of its noise occurring above the range of likely larmor frequencies. When water is cooled, or is made viscous because of dissolved substances, thermal motion slows. The magnetic fluctuations shift down into the lower frequency range, and more occur at likely resonant larmor frequencies. More stimulated emissions occur and T_1 shortens (Figure 23).

This again has a parallel in acoustics. We know from experience that audible hissing can be described as high or low. A small hole in an inflated tire produces a higher pitched hissing sound than a larger hole. Both types of hissing noise contain a wide range of frequencies, but the higher hiss contains more high-pitched frequencies than the lower hiss.

In summary, both T_1 and T_2 measure responses of hydrogen nuclei to magnetic perturbations from the environment. T_1 is solely a response to a specific frequency component in these perturbations, the resonant larmor frequency of the hydrogen nucleus. T_2 is a response to magnetic perturbations of any frequency.

Polar Macromolecules and Microviscosity

Most large molecules of biological interest are polar. Although nearly electrically neutral overall, they have an uneven distribution of charge on their surface. These local charge sites attract water molecules, which are also polar.

Because of their large size and weight, the thermal movement of macromolecules (such as proteins) is sluggish compared to that of the water in which they are dissolved. Accordingly, the thermal motion of water molecules in the vicinity of the macromolecule, or attached to its surface, is greatly slowed. We could see this effect in an ocean liner and a nearby fleet of dinghies. If a fleet of dinghies is exposed to choppy water, the small boats pitch to-and-fro in a rapid movement, whereas the motion of the ocean liner remains relatively steady. If we tied the small boats to the ocean liner, their movement would stabilize and be slowed (Figure 24).

The effect of polar macromolecules on the thermal motion of water is similar to the effect of cooling. In both cases, the motion of the water molecules is slowed and the frequencies of magnetic fluctuations produced by this motion are lowered. More magnetic fluctuations now occur at the resonant larmor frequency of the nucleus and, as a result, the rate of stimulated emission and energy loss is accelerated; T_1 is shortened.

Whether due to dissolved macromolecules or to cooling, slower thermal motion shortens T_1 of water hydrogen but has much less effect on T_2.

Paramagnetism: A Product of Orbiting Electrons

Many atoms exhibit magnetic properties which are due not to the properties of the nucleus but to the structure of their circulating clouds of electrons.

In Chapter 2, we learned a simple rule of thumb which allowed a prediction of whether or not a particular nucleus would be magnetic (Figure 6).

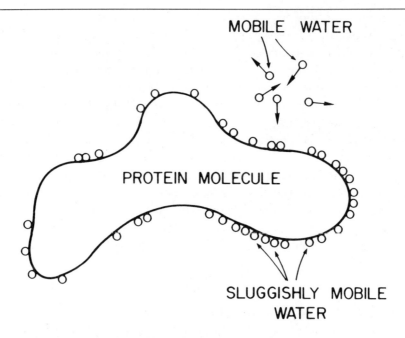

MICROVISCOSITY

Figure 24. Due to its large size, a (polar) protein molecule moves much more slowly than freely moving water molecules. Due to its polarity, it attracts the highly polar water molecules to charged sites on its surface, slowing their average motion and shortening T_1.

This magnetism resulted from the property of nuclear spin possessed by protons and neutrons. The spin of one neutron cancels the spin of its paired neutron, and similarly for protons. When the nucleus possesses an odd number of either protons or neutrons, the spin of the extra unpaired proton or neutron creates the magnetic field of the nucleus. Since the spin of a neutron cannot cancel that of a proton, if the nucleus contains both an unpaired proton and an unpaired neutron, the nucleus is still magnetic.

Electrons orbit a nucleus. This roughly circular motion of a charge produces a magnetic field in the same way that electrons moving in a circular wire produce a field. The prediction of the magnetic behavior of these orbiting electrons is complicated by the fact that, like all fundamental particles, electrons possess spin. The spin of each electron on its axis creates its own magnetic field. This magnetic effect is superimposed on that due to orbital motion, so the overall magnetic field of the electron is the sum of these two components. In some atoms, such as the noble gases, the magnetic fields from both the spin and orbital motion of the various electrons completely cancel each other, and the atom is not magnetic. In other atoms, these two factors do not cancel and consequently the atom is magnetic. These magnetic atoms are called *paramagnetic* (Figure 25).

Because of these two effects and the variable number of electrons of a

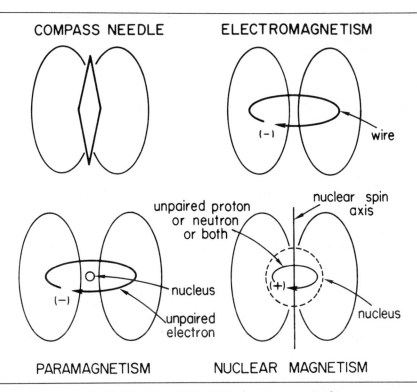

Figure 25. In Chapter 2 we learned that an atomic nucleus is magnetic if it possesses a net spin from unpaired protons or neutrons (see Figures 5 and 6). Electrons orbiting the nucleus may also produce magnetism due to their orbital motion and spin. This paramagnetism is much stronger than nuclear magnetism.

given element in various valence states, there is no simple rule allowing us to predict whether or not a given atom will be paramagnetic.

Many atoms are paramagnetic to some degree, but there is a great range. The transition elements in the middle of the periodic table show especialy strong paramagnetism. The nuclear magnetism that we have been discussing is trivial in magnitude compared to paramagnetism and can be studied only because magnetic nuclei are highly resonant at specific frequencies. It would otherwise be overshadowed by the much stronger atomic magnetism (paramagnetism) due to electrons.

The magnetism produced by the stronger paramagnetic atoms is about 1000 times greater than nuclear magnetism. As they move thermally in the microenvironment, they have powerful effects on T_1 and T_2 of hydrogen nuclei.

Ferromagnetic atoms are paramagnetic atoms which, when placed in a magnetic field, become magnetized by aligning with the external field, and which, to some degree, remain aligned and thus magnetized after the field is removed. Paramagnetic atoms also align with the field, but do not retain their alignment after removal of the field. In solution, their magnetism is important; they act as small, powerful, randomly moving magnets.

Manganese and gadolinium have been studied extensively in clinical MRI because they are strongly paramagnetic. Oxygen (O_2) in solution is also strongly paramagnetic, although the reasons for this are obscure and beyond the scope of this discussion. Fortunately, covalently-bonded oxygen, such as in water, is not paramagnetic; if it were, its strong contribution to thermal noise probably would preclude any nuclear magnetic studies of tissues.

The outer electron shells of a given element can have different numbers of electrons. These determine the valence of the atom and thus its chemical reactivity. Usually, when there is an even number of electrons in a given valence state, the atom is not paramagnetic, but an odd number of electrons in either of the outer two shells usually results in an unpaired electron, making the atom paramagnetic. For example, ferrous iron (Fe^{++}) is not paramagnetic, while ferric (Fe^{+++}) is. Gadolinium has seven unpaired electrons and, accordingly, is strongly paramagnetic. These generalizations concerning the relationship between outer shell structures and paramagnetism are not always applicable.

In solution at body temperature, paramagnetic atoms or molecules undergo the random thermal motion of other atoms and molecules. Because they are each so strongly magnetic, a very low concentration of paramagnetic atoms or molecules can have a profound effect on the much weaker magnetic nuclei of nearby atoms. They increase the magnetic white noise and intensify the fluctuations at all frequencies, including the larmor frequency. The increased fluctuations at this specific frequency trigger more T_1 decays, thereby shortening T_1.

As we have seen (Figure 22), fluctuations occurring at any frequency result in dephasing of the hydrogen nuclei. The increased magnetic noise caused by paramagnetic atoms randomly changes the field strength at nearby nuclei, resulting in more rapid dephasing and shortening of T_2. These paramagnetic effects on T_1 and T_2 are measurable even in concentrations of about one part per million.

It is difficult to determine the effects of paramagnetic substances present in the complex chemical environment of tissues. Gaseous oxygen (O_2) is present in tissues and contributes, to some undetermined extent, to a shortened T_1 and T_2. Even small amounts of artificially introduced paramagnetic substances (contrast agents) can have measurable effects on T_1 and T_2.

Gaseous oxygen has shown promise as a contrast agent; animals inhaling 100% oxygen show a detectable shortening of relaxation times in heart muscle. Manganese and gadolinium are strongly paramagnetic and have been actively studied as injectable contrast agents. These atoms can be inserted into molecules much as radioactive atoms are inserted into molecules for use in radioisotope scans in nuclear medicine. However, the chemical amounts required for MRI are much greater than those needed for radioisotope scans. Accordingly, chemical toxicity is a much greater concern. In radioactive studies, toxicity can almost always be ignored because the chemical amount of injected substance is vanishingly small. The most common paramagnetic contrast agent currently under study for use in brain is chelated gadolinium. This appears to be chemically inert and nontoxic, being excreted rapidly in the urine.

The appearance of paramagnetism in blood lying stagnant in tissues can be used to crudely estimate how long the blood has been present. Fresh blood contains hemoglobin, in which iron is in the ferrous form (Fe^{++}); it is not paramagnetic and is often difficult to differentiate from adjacent brain. After a few days at body temperature, stagnant hemoglobin is reduced to methemoglobin, in which iron is in the ferric form (Fe^{+++}) and thus paramagnetic. The corresponding shortening of relaxation times may then allow the hematoma to be differentiated from adjacent brain.

THE TERMS *LATTICE* AND *SPIN*

The interaction of excited hydrogen nuclei with their surrounding environment is usually discussed using the terms *lattice* and *spin*. To understand these terms we can consider the interaction of a water molecule with other water molecules as falling into one of two categories: interactions between a relatively few nearby nuclei and interactions between large numbers of nuclei more distant from each other. There is no sharp dividing line between those that are *nearby* and those that are *distant*.

There are relatively few molecules undergoing collisions or near-collisions with any one water molecule under examination. Consequently, the collisions and near-misses are relatively few in number, but each of these creates a strong fluctuation in local magnetic field strength.

In a larger volume surrounding the water molecule under examination, there are many more water molecules interacting from a distance. A single water molecule interacting from a distance creates a fluctuation that is relatively weak. The weak fluctuations from these many distant water molecules tend to average out since they are randomly generated; distant nuclei rarely create large fluctuations in field strength. Still, the combination of this vast number of feeble magnetic signals contains frequency components ranging from zero to billions of cycles per second (Figure 26).

NEAR ENCOUNTERS, DISTANT ENCOUNTERS: HOW THEY AFFECT T_1 AND T_2

In MRI of hydrogen nuclei, it is the motion of a nearby water molecule or paramagnetic atom that results in large fluctuations of magnetic field strength. Such large fluctuations transiently alter the resonant larmor frequencies of the nuclei under examination, causing them to become dephased from each other. We can see, then, that it is the movement of nearby magnetic particles that produces the strongest effect on T_2. This type of magnetic interaction, which occurs at short range, is called a *spin-spin* interac-

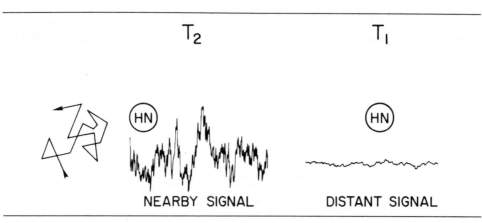

Figure 26. The thermal motion of a magnetic nucleus causes strong random fluctuations in field strength at a nearby hydrogen nucleus (HN), whose larmor frequency changes proportionately. Because the larmor frequency of each of the nuclei in a region changes randomly, they become dephased at a rate described as T_2.

At a distant nucleus, such thermal motion produces weak perturbations, which have little effect on the larmor frequency. Perturbations from trillions of other distant sources combine to create a high-frequency magnetic signal containing some component at the resonant larmor frequency, thus triggering T_1 decay.

tion. The term *spin* derives from nuclear spin, which is the basis of nuclear magnetism. The word *spin* can be interchanged with *magnet*. In *spin-spin* interaction, one magnetic nucleus is interacting directly with relatively few nearby magnetic nuclei or atoms. It could be called a one-on-one magnet-magnet interaction.

The movement of the many distant molecules creates fluctuations in magnetic field strength but, due to distance, the fluctuations are weaker than those created by nearby molecules. Because these fluctuations are weak, and because they are random (and so partially cancel, rather than reinforce each other) the interactions with distant molecules do not create the intense changes in magnetic field and resonant frequency caused by interaction with nearby water molecules. From this we can see that the interaction with distant molecules has little effect on T_2.

The many random, weak fluctuations from distant molecules create a *magnetic noise* containing a wide range of frequencies, extending both above and below likely larmor frequencies of hydrogen nuclei in MRI scanning. The small fraction of this *lattice noise* occurring at the larmor frequency has an important effect: It triggers the release of energy from stimulated nuclei, shortening T_1.

The T_1 decay of an excited magnetic nucleus in response to specific magnetic frequency components from the extended environment is traditionally called a *spin-lattice* interaction. The word *spin* again refers to the magnetic nucleus under examination. The term *lattice* refers to the extended environment of the nucleus and tends to de-emphasize the role of individual nearby nuclei in their effect on T_1. "Lattice" entered the NMR vocabulary from early studies of solids, in which the extended environment of the nucleus under examination was the orderly, repetitive pattern of atoms in a crystal lattice. Although there is no such orderly lattice structure in liquids, the term has been retained and generalized to include liquids.

We have spoken here of a few intense fluctuations originating nearby, versus a very large number of fluctuations from a distance. This could be compared to the audible noise produced from raindrops on an overhead tin roof versus all the more distant sounds of rain. The individual raindrops striking nearby cause a few discrete, loud sounds. Each raindrop is perceived as an individual event. This is analogous to the few large fluctuations caused by thermal noise originating nearby (the basis of T_2). The sound of distant rain is produced by very many raindrops, each of which is too distant to be audible individually, and which together create a constant hissing sound similar to that of steam escaping. This is analogous to lattice magnetic noise stimulating T_1 relaxation.

T_1 AND T_2 IN TISSUES

Each of the factors mentioned above — temperature, paramagnetism, polar macromolecules — changes thermal motion and so alters the magnetic environment of the hydrogen nucleus we are imaging by MRI. In a laboratory situation, using an NMR relaxation analyzer, it is possible to study in isolation the effect of each of these factors on the behavior (relaxation times) of the hydrogen nucleus.

Starting with a sample of pure water (in which T_1 and T_2 are both about 2.7 seconds), we can lower the temperature, add an amount of protein, or add a paramagnetic substance, and then measure the exact changes in T_1 and T_2 independently of each other. Each of the above three factors shortens T_1. Paramagnetic substances shorten both T_1 and T_2, while adding large molecules or cooling has little effect on T_2. (Temperature is not a significant factor in MRI, because the internal temperature of humans is quite constant.)

In vitro NMR analysis of a complex mixture can be performed and T_1 and T_2 measured with considerable accuracy, provided the sample is large enough to be measured, is homogeneous, and enough analysis time is allocated.

Measuring the relaxation times of living tissues using MRI differs substantially from laboratory measurement of simple solutions. First, tissue fluids are very complex mixtures of macromolecules and paramagnetic substances; the exact composition of tissue fluids at any one moment cannot be determined.

In pure water, T_1 and T_2 are about equal (2.7 seconds). In tissues, T_1 and T_2 are shorter: T_1 is about one fifth that of pure water, while T_2 is about one fiftieth. This shortening of T_1 and T_2 relative to pure water is due to the increased viscosity of tissue water and the presence of paramagnetic substances. The reason for the greater shortening of T_2 relative to T_1 is not clear but may be because, magnetically, many cellular components behave as though they were somewhere between a liquid and a solid. In true solids, T_2 is very much shorter than T_1, and T_1 is greatly prolonged. The semisolid state of much of the tissue hydrogen may explain the absolute T_1 and T_2 observed in tissues. In pathology, changes in the nature of this semisolid state may explain many of the changes in relaxation.

Each substance dissolved in tissue water wields its own influence on the behavior of the hydrogen nuclei in the water molecules. The complicated interrelationships between tissue components and their effects on relaxation times are now under intensive study; much useful data can be expected within the next decade.

Compartmentalization

Another way that T_1 and T_2 measurements of living tissue differ from laboratory measurements is lack of homogeneity: Except for a few anatomical compartments, such as the cerebral ventricles, amniotic fluid, urinary bladder, cysts, and major vascular channels, large volumes of homogeneous fluid do not occur in the normal body. In living tissues, there is a very complex assemblage of macromolecules, lipoprotein membranes, various intracellular microscopic structures, and paramagnetic substances, which are not homogeneously distributed. Probably, various submicroscopic cellular compartments have widely differing T_1's and T_2's.

Each of the thousands of pixels (picture elements) that make up an MRI scan represents a composite of T_1, T_2, and hydrogen distribution within a volume element (voxel). Scanning can be weighted to emphasize any one, or a combination, of these factors. Typical dimensions of a voxel might be $1 \times 1 \times 10$ millimeters. Within this voxel might be several hundred thousand cells, each with subcompartments having their own T_1 and T_2. Surrounding the cells is a thin layer of extracellular fluid, whose composition (and therefore T_1 and T_2) is much closer to that of pure water than is intracellular fluid. For the entire body, extracellular fluid makes up an average of 20% of the total tissue volume. When MRI of living tissues is performed, the signal from the layer of extracellular fluid surrounding the cells is averaged by the scanner with the signal from the intracellular water and various cellular subcompartments, and some composite value results.

Each cell has an endoplasmic reticulum, an extensive labyrinth of proteolipid membrane which has an enormous surface area. Such extensive, relatively stiff, semifluid structures probably slow the movement of adjacent water in the cell cytoplasm and so shorten T_1, for the same reasons as macromolecules. Similarly, mitochondria, each possessing a large area of interfolding membranes, fill up 10% to 30% of most cells. Both of these highly membranous subcompartments have their own structural and chemical characteristics, and probably distinctive values for T_1 and T_2. In liver cells, endoplasmic reticulum and mitochondrial membranes account for 90% of total tissue membrane (Blouin *et al*, in Fawcett, 1981).

It will be fascinating to learn, over the next few years, how microscopic changes in cell membranous structure affect relaxation times in various pathologies.

RELAXATION TIME ACCURACY

In the MRI scanner, it is difficult to take a large enough number of measurements to provide accurate T_1 and T_2 values, because of the practical limitations on the length of time the patient can be expected to lie motionless in the center of the long tube of the MRI gantry. It is difficult to extrapolate from any two or three image data points to predict accurate relaxation times. It would be much more accurate if 20 or 30 data points could be obtained. This is practical in the laboratory but not in the clinical setting. In addition to inconsistencies from a single MRI scanner, relaxation times seem to differ substantially from machine to machine. Greater relaxation time accuracy will undoubtedly be realized in the future.

It is impossible to determine from scans that display T_1 or T_2 just what complex chemical or structural factors have contributed to these relaxation times. In clinical use of MRI, correlations between pathology and T_1 and T_2 are presently established empirically. For example, while it is known that most types of brain pathological lesions lengthen T_2, and so are seen best by T_2-weighted scans, the exact reasons for this are not known.

Since MRI observes hydrogen nuclei and changes in their behavior, it cannot directly observe the macromolecules or paramagnetic substances that cause the environmental changes. All that can be measured in a T_1- or T_2-weighted scan is the total change in the magnetic environment affecting either of these two factors.

To return to the analogy with which we opened this chapter, we can again compare magnetic resonance imaging of hydrogen nuclei to the observation of people on the street below a hotel room window. We know a great deal about human response to weather because of extended, detailed observation. We know very little about the behavioral responses of tissue water to different pathophysiological circumstances because we have relatively little experience. It is to be hoped that we will become as familiar with these tissue interrelationships as we are with people responding to the weather.

PULSE SEQUENCING

Our knowledge of the tissues is derived from the brief signal re-emitted from the tissues after the stimulating pulse. Since both T_1 and T_2 cause the duration of this signal to shorten, how is it possible to distinguish their relative contributions and produce scans emphasizing either T_1 or T_2?

With the approach to imaging we have described so far — using a single stimulating pulse — it is impossible to separate the effects of T_1 and T_2. A single pulse can give us mainly regional hydrogen concentration. To measure T_1 and T_2, the stimulation of the tissues is modified. Instead of one pulse of radio-frequency energy, two or more pulses are applied in quick succession.

Such pulse sequences cause the re-emitted signal to contain extractable information about T_1 and T_2.

By changing the parameters of the pulse sequence — number of pulses, strengths of the pulses, time intervals between the pulses — different types of information can be elicited from the tissues. The MRI scan can be weighted to emphasize information about T_1, T_2, or hydrogen distribution.

When a slice of tissue is scanned using various pulse sequences, such as spinecho or inversion-recovery, the resulting scans can appear dramatically different. It is as though they were made from large tissue slices actually cut from the organ and stained by various histological techniques.

These different pulse sequences are the imaging strategies referred to in the Introduction. For the interested reader, they will be expanded upon in Chapter 5.

CHAPTER 5: TISSUE CHARACTERIZATION AND PULSE SEQUENCING

In preceding chapters, we described the physics of MRI using a classical approach. We started by comparing the properties of a hydrogen nucleus with those of a more familiar object — a compass needle. This comparison was valid because a compass needle and a hydrogen nucleus share several properties: In the presence of a magnetic field, they both tend to align with the external field, absorb energy through the phenomenon of resonance, and subsequently re-emit this energy. Each oscillates at a frequency that is proportional to the strength of the magnetic field. In the case of the hydrogen nucleus, this oscillatory frequency is the resonant (or larmor) frequency.

To develop a deeper understanding of MRI, particularly of tissue characterization and pulse-sequencing, we need to develop a more precise description of nuclear behavior. It would seem logical to start with the study of an individual hydrogen nucleus, just as we started our earlier explanations with the behavior of an individual compass needle. However, the detailed description of the behavior of an individual hydrogen nucleus, trillions of times as small as a compass needle, is extremely complex. Such detailed descriptions require a knowledge of quantum physics and are therefore beyond the scope of this book. (An introduction to quantum principles in MRI is contained in the Appendix.)

Fortunately, it is unnecessary to understand the behavior of a single nucleus to understand MRI. It is impossible to observe a single nucleus: The signal it generates is much too weak to be measured. What is observed,

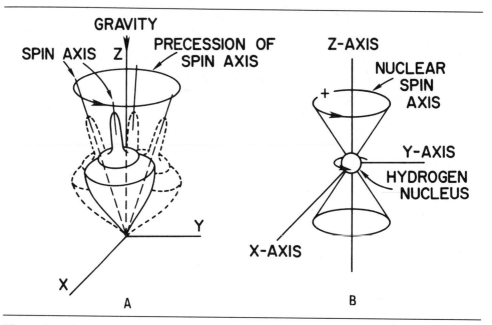

Figure 27. The toy top (A) spins about its own axis, which precesses in the Earth's gravitational field. The hydrogen nucleus (B) possesses nuclear spin; its spin axis precesses in the magnetic field of the scanner.

rather, is the aggregate signal from many billions of nuclei. Although individually they follow quantum laws, the collective behavior of the nuclei and the signal they produce can be described in classical terms. The aggregate response of the hydrogen nuclei in the few cubic millimeters of tissue in a voxel is, in many respects, remarkably like one large compass needle.

In modern science, there are many other examples of a knowledge of the fine details of a process not being necessary for it to be exploited. A satellite may be put in orbit without any application of the theory of relativity, because the effects of relativity in this particular situation are trivial. Similarly, a motion picture director produces as a final product a developed piece of photographic film, but need know nothing about the chemistry of the photographic process.

In this chapter, we will discuss the classical description of nuclear behavior and then apply it to imaging, pulse-sequencing, and T_1- and T_2-weighting of MRI scans.

Before going on to describe collective behavior, we will make one further comparison between the individual nucleus and the compass needle: their manner of oscillation. Because its movement is restricted by a fixed bearing, a compass needle oscillates in a single plane. The hydrogen nucleus, in three-dimensional space, oscillates in a wobbling motion about the direction of the magnetic field. This type of motion is called *precession* and is familiar to us as the wobbling motion of a spinning toy top in the Earth's gravitational field. The number of times per second that the nucleus wobbles or precesses is its resonant frequency (Figure 27).

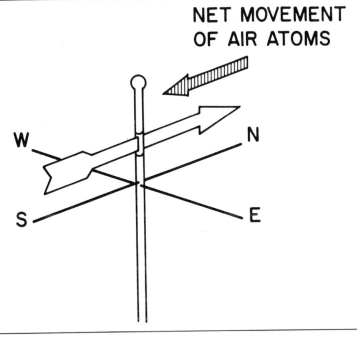

NET MOVEMENT OF AIR ATOMS

Figure 28. A weather vane indicates the net movement of air molecules, even though they are all moving randomly at about the speed of sound. In tissues, the magnetization vector represents the net behavior of the nuclei in the randomly moving molecules; the nuclei tend to align with the scanner's magnetic field.

THE MAGNETIZATION VECTOR

To describe the behavior of hydrogen nuclei during MRI, we use an imaginary construct: the magnetization vector, a single vector which represents the aggregate behavior of all hydrogen nuclei in a small region of tissue. While most texts describe the magnetization vector for an infinitely small region of tissue, for convenience, we will say that this small region is a voxel, the volume element of tissue being imaged. The magnetization vector is described using a coordinate system whose X-, Y-, and Z-axes coincide with those of the scanner's magnetic field and whose origin is in the middle of the voxel of tissue being imaged. The tail of the vector is fixed at this origin, and its length and direction at any moment express the overall behavior of the hydrogen nuclei in the voxel.

The magnetization vector may usefully be compared to a weather vane. Air atoms move with a frenetic random motion, at about the speed of sound. Many millions of air molecules strike the weather vane each second. In still air, the number of such impacts on all surfaces of the vane is nearly constant; they cancel each other, and the vane points in no particular direction. In addition to this random motion, the atoms may exhibit a much slower net motion in a particular direction (the wind). The weather vane expresses this net motion and ignores the random. From moment to moment, the direction of the weather vane changes to reflect changes in the wind (Figure 28).

Similarly, in tissues there is a very large number of water molecules undergoing random thermal motion. In MRI, the nuclei are exposed to both constant magnetic fields and to intermittent radio energy. When the nuclei are exposed to a constant magnetic field, they have a small net tendency to align with this field; when exposed to radio energy, they have a small net tendency to be driven away from alignment. The magnetization vector expresses this average magnetic orientation of the nuclei in the voxel under examination, in response to these influences. When there is no external magnetic field, the nuclear orientations are randomly directed, much as the movement of air molecules in still air.

This vector allows us to make the conceptual leap from the magnetic resonance of a compass needle to the aggregate behavior of many magnetic nuclei in tissues. Although individually, nuclei must be described by quantum physics, their aggregate behavior can be expressed by the magnetization vector, which is described classically, in a manner more analogous to a compass needle. For teaching purposes, we can substitute the magnetization vector for the compass needle in many of our earlier explanations (Figure 29).

General Behavior of Magnetization Vector

We can discuss, in a general manner, the behavior of the magnetization vector during the MRI scan process: alignment before stimulation, stimulation by RF energy, oscillation, and subsequent loss of energy.

When a patient is placed in the strong magnetic field of an MRI scanner, hydrogen nuclei in the tissues tend to align themselves with the field. The magnetization vector reflects this by aligning with the main field of the scanner (along the positive Z-axis). The length of the vector is proportional to the number of nuclei in the voxel and to the applied magnetic field strength. Exposure of the voxel of tissue to radio-frequency energy (at the larmor frequency) results in the nuclei absorbing energy, and a tendency for them to be deflected away from alignment; the magnetization vector is deflected so that it tilts away from the direction of the main field. Just as the angle to which a compass needle is deflected depends on how hard it has been tapped, so too the angle to which the magnetization vector tilts is proportional to the strength of the radio-frequency pulse.

Once energized, the tilted magnetization vector precesses about the Z-axis at the larmor frequency, representing an extremely large number of individually precessing nuclei. As the nuclei lose energy, the angle that the precessing magnetization vector makes with the main field diminishes; eventually the vector comes back to rest aligned with the main field.

For the purposes of MRI, the magnetization vector can be treated as if it were a real magnet. When a real magnet moves in relation to a stationary antenna coil, its lines of magnetic force cut through the coil, inducing a voltage. In MRI, the magnetization vector is at rest before stimulation, lying along the positive Z-axis, and induces no voltage in the antenna coil. After

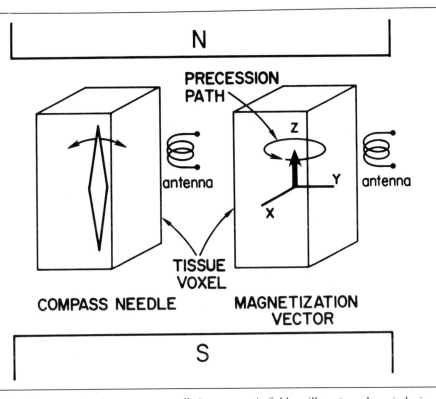

Figure 29. When energized, a compass needle in a magnetic field oscillates in a plane, inducing a signal in an antenna coil.

The magnetic behavior of the many hydrogen nuclei in a voxel of tissue can be represented by a single arrow, the magnetization vector. In many ways, this vector behaves as if it were a real bar magnet, such as a compass needle. When it absorbs energy, it oscillates in a precessional motion about the Z-axis, inducing a signal in the antenna.

stimulation, it precesses and so induces in the antenna of the MRI scanner a signal that oscillates at the larmor frequency.

In the imaging process, all the voxels in the slice of tissue being imaged are stimulated: The magnetization vector for each voxel is tipped away from the Z-axis by the same angle. Initially, the vectors all precess at the same larmor frequency. However, to furthur localize the voxels, the scanner applies a new gradient transversely across the slice, slightly raising or lowering the magnetic field at various locations in the slice. In response, the larmor frequency of the magnetization vector for each voxel changes accordingly. Vectors at different locations in the slice induce signals of different frequencies in the antenna. The position of a voxel in the gradient can thus be deduced from the frequency of its signal.

A recognition of this immediate responsiveness of the magnetization vector to changes in local field strength following excitation is crucial to the understanding of MRI.

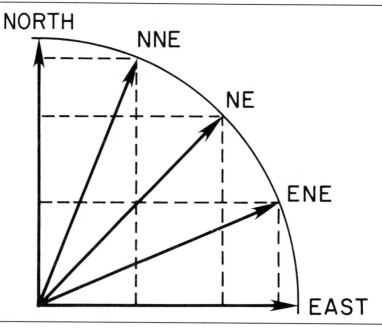

Figure 30. A single vector can be expressed as the sum of two (or three) vectors. For example, the points of a compass can be expressed as the sum of any two cardinal directions. Northeast, for instance, is the sum of equal-lengthed vectors pointing in the north and east directions.

In the next section, we will analyze the magnetization vector in more detail. This analysis will provide insight into T_1, T_2, and signal strength.

COMPONENT VECTORS

Most mathematical descriptions of a vector in three-dimensional space describe the vector as a sum of three component vectors, one for each of the coordinate axes — X, Y, and Z. By summing the components lying along each of the axes, a vector of any length and orientation can be obtained. A simple example of the addition of vectors is the points of a compass (Figure 30).

In MRI, it is convenient to describe the magnetization vector in terms of only two component vectors. One vector lies on the Z-axis, paralleling the main field. The second vector lies in the plane defined by the X- and Y-axes, at right angles to the main field (Figure 31). This second vector could be further resolved as the sum of vectors along the X- and Y-axes, similar to compass points. Since the main field in most scanners is longitudinal, the Z-axis component is usually referred to as the longitudinal component, while the vector in the X-Y plane is the transverse component. (By convention, Y is front-to-back of the patient, X is left-to-right of the patient.)

The importance of the components of the magnetization vector is that each is related to an aspect of nuclear behavior: The longitudinal component is

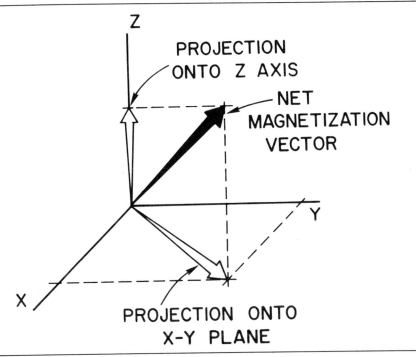

Figure 31. The length of the magnetization vector is proportional to the number of hydrogen nuclei in the voxel. At any moment during imaging, the direction of the vector indicates the average position of these nuclei. Here the magnetization vector is shown tipped 45° from the Z-axis, toward the X-Y plane. Its longitudinal and transverse projections (onto the Z-axis and the X-Y plane respectively) are equal.

related to T_1 and the transverse component to T_2. We will see that the transverse component is also related to signal strength.

Components of Magnetization Vector after Stimulation

With these simple tools, we can describe in a more precise manner the response of the magnetization vector to a radio-frequency pulse.

Before stimulation, the magnetization vector is entirely longitudinal, being aligned with the main field along the positive Z-axis. It is stationary, has no transverse component, and produces no signal.

Upon stimulation, the magnetization vector is driven from the positive Z-axis some number of degrees, depending on the strength of the pulse. The strength of the pulse is indicated by the number of degrees it deflects the magnetization vector. Because the length of the vector is the same immediately after stimulation as before, the exact angle of the magnetization vector determines the initial values of the longitudinal and transverse components. With a relatively short (weak) pulse, the vector might be deflected 10°; as a result, the longitudinal vector is shortened slightly, while the transverse vector attains a measurable value.

One might imagine the Z-axis component of the vector by visualizing the shadow cast on it from a light source located on the Y-axis, in the transverse plane. The vector projection on the X-Y plane could similarly be imagined by considering the vector's shadow cast on the plane from a light source located on the Z-axis, above the transverse plane.

As pulse strength increases from zero to 90°, the longitudinal component shortens, while the transverse component grows. A 90° pulse places the magnetization vector entirely in the transverse plane, producing the maximum length of the transverse component. Increasing pulse lengths from 90° to 180° results in a shorter transverse component but in a longitudinal component that is longer in the negative (downward) Z-axis direction. At 180°, the longitudinal component achieves a maximum negative value, while the transverse component becomes zero. Still stronger pulses drive the magnetization vector beyond 180°, producing a longitudinal component that is shorter in the negative Z-direction, but a transverse component that is larger. At 270°, the longitudinal component is zero, while the transverse component is again maximal. Similarly, pulses between 270° and 360° produce longitudinal components that are longer in the positive Z-direction, and transverse components that again shorten. At 360°, the magnetization vector is driven completely around a circle, coming to rest in the positive Z direction, in its pre-stimulation state.

With the exception of 180° and 360° pulses (which place the magnetization vector along the negative and positive Z-axis, respectively), the magnetization vector is tilted away from the Z-axis and precesses at the larmor frequency.

Transverse Component and Signal Strength

There are several reasons to analyze the magnetization vector in terms of its component vectors. The first of these concerns signal strength.

Earlier we stated that the precessing magnetization vector induces a measurable signal in the antenna coil. The antenna of the MRI scanner consists essentially of a pair of coils of wire lying perpendicular to the X-Y plane. Only the component of precessional motion which is at right angles to the antenna (i.e., the transverse component) can induce this voltage. Therefore, the signal strength from a voxel is proportional to the length of the transverse component.

We saw earlier that the stimulating radio frequency pulse drives the magnetization vectors for all the voxels in the slice of tissue being imaged to approximately the same angle, at which they precess at a larmor frequency appropriate to their position in the transverse gradient. We know that the length of an individual magnetization vector depends on the number of hydrogen nuclei in its voxel. The more nuclei in a voxel, the longer its magnetization vector; the longer the transverse component, the stronger the signal from that voxel.

The antenna measures the signal from a slice of tissue after a single excitation pulse; in the presence of a transverse gradient, it receives signals at many slightly different frequencies. Each frequency component of this signal corresponds to the position of a line across the slice of tissue in the gradient. The strength of the signal at that frequency indicates the number of nuclei in the cross section at that position (see Chapter 3).

Component Vectors and Tissue Characterization

The initial length of the transverse component (and the initial signal strength from a voxel) is an indication of regional tissue hydrogen concentration. But in MRI, we are interested in tissue characterization beyond simple hydrogen concentration: specifically, the rate at which nuclei lose energy (T_1) and the rate at which nuclei become dephased (T_2). To determine T_1 and T_2, we will examine the behavior of the magnetization vector's components after stimulation, as the nuclei relax back to their prestimulation state. To analyze T_1, we will examine how the longitudinal component changes; to analyze T_2, we will examine the behavior of the transverse component.

BEHAVIOR OF LONGITUDINAL AND TRANSVERSE COMPONENTS

While the above discussion focused mainly on the initial lengths of the transverse and longitudinal vectors immediately after stimulation, it is the subsequent behavior of these vectors — how they change after stimulation — that reflects tissue characteristics.

In the next section, we consider the behavior of the longitudinal and transverse components as expressions of T_1 and T_2.

Because T_1 and T_2 are largely independent processes, we must learn to conceptualize the behavior of the longitudinal and transverse components of the magnetization vector separately. We can then use these component vectors to compare the rates T_1 and T_2 and to relate these relaxation processes to signal strength.

Longitudinal Component and T_1

The longitudinal vector is related to the energy of the excited nuclei in the voxel; the rate at which the longitudinal vector changes length after stimulation expresses how rapidly energy is lost from the nuclei (this is expressed as the time constant T_1).

Before stimulation, the magnetization vector is entirely longitudinal, lying at rest along the positive Z-axis. As stated, the initial length of the longitudinal component after stimulation is related to the angle to which the magnetization vector is driven, which in turn is related to the amount of energy in the stimulating pulse: The longitudinal component takes on some value between its original extreme length in the positive (up) Z direction and the same length in the negative (down) Z direction. (In Figure 32, the magnetization vector is shown before and after a 180° pulse.)

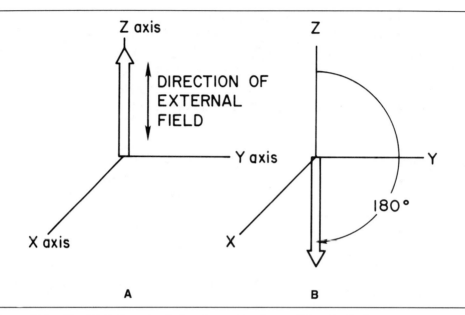

Figure 32A + B. (A) Before stimulation the positive (upward) longitudinal component is maximal.
(B) After a 180° pulse, the longitudinal component has the same length but lies along the negative (downward) Z-axis.

After stimulation, the nuclei start to lose their energy; the longitudinal component starts to grow back in the positive Z direction. The rate of energy loss — and the rate at which the longitudinal component grows — is determined by T_1. No matter what its initial length and orientation (whether directed along the positive or negative Z-axes), after stimulation the transverse component starts to grow back in the positive Z direction at rate T_1 (Figure 33).

The upward growth of the longitudinal component (and T_1 energy loss) cannot be measured directly but has an important effect on the spin–echo pulse sequence; it can also be measured by the inversion–recovery pulse sequence. Both are described later in this chapter.

The more energy that is contained in the stimulating radio pulse, the larger the angle the magnetization vector is moved through. As pulse strength increases from zero to 180°, the longitudinal component becomes longer in the negative Z direction, and it takes longer for the longitudinal component to return to its original positive Z orientation. So far, this seems logical: The more energy is pumped into the tissues, the longer it takes for the longitudinal component to return to equilibrium. However, at pulses stronger than 180°, the relationship between the energizing pulse and the longitudinal component becomes counter-intuitive: The pulses contain more energy, but result in a longitudinal component that is shorter and which takes less time to grow back to its prestimulation state.

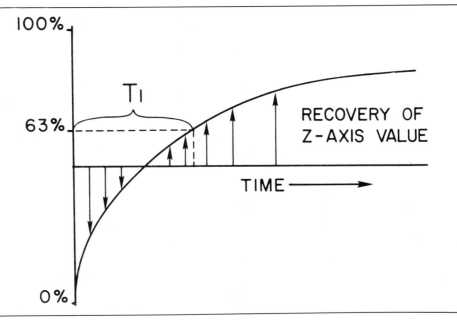

Figure 33. The growth of the longitudinal component after a 180° pulse is shown. After a stimulating pulse, the nuclei undergo T_1 relaxation (energy loss) at an exponential rate. T_1 is defined as the time it takes for the longitudinal component to regain 63% of its length.

Transverse Component

Because it is precessing at the larmor frequency, the transverse component is an expression of the precessional motion of the many nuclei within the voxel. The length of the transverse component at any moment after stimulation is an expression of the phase coherence between the nuclei, that is, how well their phases are locked together.

The stimulating radio frequency pulse locks in phase the precessional motions of the nuclei in the voxel: Immediately after excitation, the transverse component of the magnetization vector has a maximum length and is precessing at the larmor frequency. Although the nuclei are initially locked in phase by the stimulating pulse, local magnetic forces in the tissue cause fluctuations in the precessional rate of individual nuclei: The nuclei quickly become dephased. As they become randomly phased, the nuclei cancel each other's magnetic effects: The transverse component shrinks and disappears. Because it is both shortening and rotating, the tip of the transverse component describes an ever-narrowing spiral. When the nuclei are completely dephased, the transverse component is zero.

The rate at which the transverse component changes length expresses the rate of dephasing.

Sources of dephasing

There are two important causes of dephasing. The first, T_2 from thermal motion in tissues, was discussed in Chapter 4 because it is important in characterizing tissues. The second, nonuniformity of field strength, is actually the major source of dephasing in MRI. Due to inevitable variations in the scanner's magnetic field, tissue magnetic properties, and applied gradient fields, there are slight but important variations in field strength from point to point within the volume being imaged. These nonuniformities are fundamentally different from those that occur on the molecular level, due to thermal motion, which were described in Chapter 4. The term for dephasing due to fixed distortions of the field is T_2-star, which, although it does not reflect tissue characteristics, nonetheless plays an important part in the imaging process.

No magnet can produce a perfectly uniform magnetic field. Although the magnets used in MRI create magnetic fields that are extremely uniform (from one part in ten thousand to one in a million), even such slight imperfections can have striking effects. Two adjacent anatomical regions may differ in field strength by only one part in a million, but if their precessional frequency is 50 million cycles per second, they will drift 180° out of phase in 10 milliseconds. This indicates the inevitability of the effects of field nonuniformity.

The field of the scanner is also distorted by the presence of the patient's body, which has very weak magnetic properties. To understand this, we can think how a piece of iron placed in a uniform magnetic field will attract and concentrate the magnetic field within itself, causing the field strength there to be much greater than elsewhere. This ability to concentrate magnetic field is known as *magnetic susceptibility*. To a much less striking degree than iron, various regions of tissue have varying magnetic susceptibility, resulting in different field strengths within an initially uniform field. This can come, for example, from paramagnetic atoms found in varying amounts in the tissues. In the presence of the scanner's magnetic field, these become aligned and cause a slight, unpredictable regional concentration of the main field.

In addition to these uncontrollable nonuniformities, there is the intentionally created nonuniformity due to the magnetic gradients. In our explanations up to now, we have assumed that an individual voxel is exposed to a uniform field. In fact, the gradient creates a differential magnetic field across the voxel.

In practice, the gradient magnetic fields usually are the strongest of these three sources of dephasing. All three of these sources of nonuniformity of field are constant over time and cause the larmor frequency to vary slightly in different regions of the field. As a result, the precessional phase relationships of the nuclei drift apart in a constant and predictable manner.

The dephasing of hydrogen nuclei, then, comes from these constant sources of nonuniformity, as well as from the fluctuating nonuniformities due to tissue random thermal magnetic noise. In practice, the dephasing caused by constant nonuniformities of field (T_2-star) contributes much more dephasing than that caused by thermal noise (T_2).

There is an important difference between the dephasing produced by T_2 and that produced by T_2-star: Nuclei in regions whose nonuniformities are constant go out of phase with each other at a constant rate (T_2-star), but random fluctuations from thermal noise cause nuclei to go out of phase randomly (T_2).

Dephasing and signal strength

Immediately after excitation, the transverse component of the magnetization vector is long, signifying that the precessional phase coherence is high: Precessions are not cancelling other (nearby) precessions, but instead reinforce each other, so the received radio signal is strong. As the nuclei go out of phase, the transverse component shortens and the signal weakens.

Whereas the initial amplitude of the signal is a measure of hydrogen concentration, the rate of decay of the signal indicates rate of dephasing due to T_2 and T_2-star.

ROTATING FRAME OF REFERENCE

Until now, we have been observing the motion of the transverse component from a stationary external point of view. We see it rotating at the larmor frequency about the Z-axis as it shortens (due to dephasing). To simplify analysis of this behavior, it is common to imagine that the point of view of the observer is some distance above the transverse plane, on the Z-axis, and rotating at approximately the larmor frequency. This is called the *rotating frame of reference*.

Because our frame of reference is rotating with the transverse component, the magnetization vector lying in the transverse plane appears to stop, and minor changes in phase relationships can be observed with great precision. When using the magnetization vector to describe nuclear behavior, it is necessary to specify whether the frame of reference is external (stationary) or rotating (Figure 34).

This means of examining rotating objects could be illustrated by a merry-go-round. If we stand outside the merry-go-round and observe its motion, as the various horses and other objects blur past us, we could not hope to distinguish any of their details. However, if we climbed to the top and looked through a hole on the axis of rotation, we would be turning with the entire array of horses and passengers; each of them would now seem to be nearly stationary, and we could tell one horse from another and even recognize passengers. By rotating with this complicated machine, we place ourselves in its frame of reference.

We will examine the effect of a pulse on the magnetization vector, and the subsequent behavior of the vector, as viewed from a rotating frame of reference. We need to point out two facts about radio-pulse/tissue interaction. First, in MRI, radio frequency pulses arrive from a specific direction (usually along the X-axis) and are not simply beamed into the tissues from all sides. Second, when the magnetization vector is deflected by the pulse, it tends to align perpendicular to the direction of the radio-frequency pulse.

Consider a 90° pulse entering the tissues in the transverse plane along the

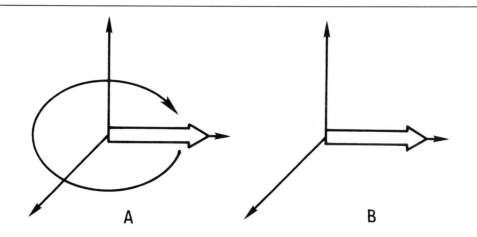

Figure 34A + B. (A) The magnetization vector after a 90° pulse, as viewed from an external frame. The vector lies in the transverse plane and rotates at the larmor frequency.
(B) The magnetization vector after a 90° pulse, as viewed from a rotating frame. The vector appears to lie still in the transverse plane. It is easier to ι ε the magnetization vector in the rotating frame to describe subtle changes in subsequent precessional motion.

X-axis. The magnetization vector, which is originally aligned with the positive Z-axis, is deflected 90° into the X-Y plane and lies along the Y-axis (or perpendicular to the direction of origin of the pulse). Initially, the transverse magnetization vector appears as a single vector, because the nuclei are in phase. Because we are rotating with it (at the larmor frequency) it lies stationary on the Y-axis. As time passes and the precessional rates of nuclei change, we observe the transverse component dispersing into many shorter vectors in the X-Y plane, fanning out clockwise and counter clockwise away from the original Y-axis transverse component, expressing the fact that nuclei are ahead or behind in phase (Figure 35).

In this rotating frame of reference, we could also distinguish the two sources of dephasing: that due to constant local field nonuniformities (T_2-star) and that due to randomly changing thermal motion (T_2): The vectors representing T_2-star dephasing fan out at constant rates, while those representing T_2 dephasing spread out randomly.

COMPARING THE LONGITUDINAL AND TRANSVERSE COMPONENTS
In summary, the magnetization vector expresses, in a single arrow, the average behavior of hydrogen in a region of tissue. By noting its projections onto the longitudinal Z-axis or onto the transverse X-Y plane, we can examine more specific behavior: The changing projection on the Z-axis describes T_1 relaxation; the shrinking projection on the X-Y plane describes T_2 and T_2-star relaxation.

We will consider the stimulation of nuclei in a voxel by a 90° pulse, using

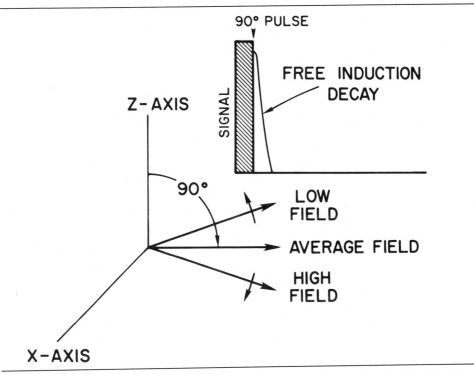

Figure 35. Immediately after the stimulating pulse, the nuclei are precessing in phase. But due to nonuniformities in the field, they precess at different rates, becoming progressively dephased. As seen in the rotating frame, the transverse component disperses into many vectors, which spread clockwise and counterclockwise in the X-Y plane.

the longitudinal and transverse components to compare the rates of energy loss and dephasing, and correlate this behavior with the measured signal.

Before stimulation, the magnetization vector is entirely longitudinal, has a finite value, and points upward along the positive Z-axis; the transverse component is zero. In this unstimulated equilibrium state, there is no signal being produced. The 90° pulse drives the magnetization vector 90° into the transverse plane, putting the precessions of the nuclei into phase with each other. The longitudinal component is zero immediately after this stimulation, but the length of the transverse component is maximal, and it rotates in the X-Y plane at the larmor frequency (as viewed from the stationary external frame of reference), thereby inducing a signal in the antenna coil (Figure 36).

The nuclei immediately begin to lose their energy (due to T_1), and their precessional motions start to become dephased (due to T_2 and T_2-star); the longitudinal component begins to grow in the positive Z direction, while at the same time the transverse component begins to shrink towards zero (Figure 37).

In tissues, dephasing occurs much more rapidly than T_1 energy loss: T_1 is between 150 and 2000 milliseconds, T_2 is 20 to 120 milliseconds, while

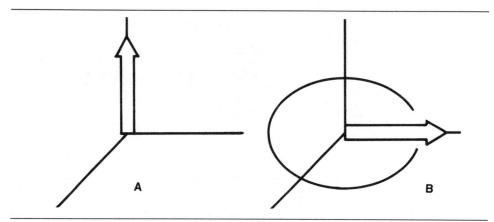

Figure 36A + B. (A) A 90° pulse tilts the magnetization vector from its original longitudinal orientation into the transverse plane.
(B) In a stationary frame, the magnetization vector rotates in the transverse plane at the larmor frequency.

T_2-star is 1 to 10 milliseconds. Consequently, the transverse component under the influence of T_2-star shortens faster than the longitudinal component grows, diminishing to zero in 1 to 10 milliseconds, long before the longitudinal component regains its original length. The loss of signal is correspondingly rapid, due primarily to dephasing.

When the transverse component reaches zero, the longitudinal component has regained only a fraction of its original length. The longitudinal component continues to grow, at a rate T_1, until it reaches it original (prestimulation) length and orientation.

This fact — that the signal falls to zero long before T_1 energy loss is complete — will be of importance in discussions of the spin-echo pulse sequence (later in this chapter) and of scan time (in Chapter 8).

PULSE STRENGTH, SIGNAL STRENGTH, AND SIGNAL LOSS

We wish to measure T_1 and T_2, but using a single pulse, T_1 is impossible to measure because the longitudinal component produces no signal. Similarly, T_2 alone cannot be measured, because its dephasing effects are combined with those of T_2-star, causing signal loss.

To measure T_1 or T_2 alone, we must use pulse sequencing, a series of several pulses. Before discussing pulse sequencing, however, we must consider in more detail the relationships between tissue response and the single radio-frequency pulse discussed in the previous sections. Specifically, we will investigate the relationships between pulse strength, signal strength, and signal loss.

Apparatus

To simplify our analysis, we will use a simple apparatus similar to that used by Bloch and Purcell to demonstrate the phenomenon of NMR in 1946. It

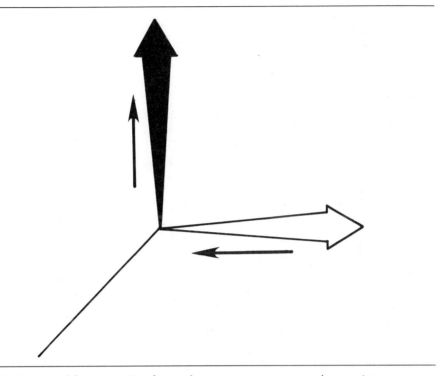

Figure 37. As viewed from a rotating frame, the transverse component shortens (at a rate determined by dephasing), and the longitudinal component grows (at a rate determined by energetic loss). Dephasing occurs more rapidly than energetic loss, so shortening of the transverse component occurs more rapidly than growth of the longitudinal component. As the transverse component shortens, the detected signal decays. The black arrow shows the final equilibrium position of the vector after complete relaxation.

consists of a strong permanent magnet between whose pole faces is suspended a small test tube, which contains a small sample representing our tissue voxel. Around this test tube there are two loops of wire: One loop transmits the stimulating radio signal into the sample; the other loop is an antenna measuring the subsequent signal-out from the sample (Figure 38). By connecting the antenna to a radio receiver and displaying the output signal on an oscilloscope, we can observe in detail the answer to each question: the shape and amplitude of the emitted signal.

In these experiments, the sample is exposed to a uniform field, so that all the hydrogens in the sample experience approximately the same field strength and have the same larmor frequency. If the test tube is exposed to a one tesla field, the resonant larmor frequency of the hydrogen in the sample is 42.6 million cycles per second. In the following basic experiments, the radio signal used to stimulate the sample has this frequency.

The sample in the test tube is blood serum, which is almost entirely water (and it is this water we are analyzing). Various dissolved substances cause it to behave quite differently from pure water and more like tissue.

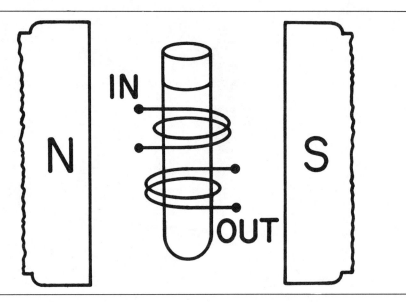

Figure 38. To demonstrate the response of a tissue sample to magnetic interrogation, only a simple apparatus is needed. A test tube is placed between the poles of a magnet. Two loops of wire encircle the test tube, one transmitting a short burst of radio-frequency energy into the sample, the other acting as an antenna which listens to the signal emitted by the sample (blood serum).

Signal Loss — The Free Induction Decay

In this experiment, we expose the test tube sample to a single pulse and observe the re-emitted signal immediately after the pulse. If the pulse length is 180° or 360°, there will be no measurable signal (because there is no transverse component). However after pulses of other lengths, there is a transverse component, and a signal can be detected; the sample re-emits the energy in a smoothly-decaying signal. This signal is the free induction decay.

This brief decaying signal is the sole source of information from which images can be constructed.

In this example, we are not interested in the initial amplitude of the signal from the tissues, but in the shape of the curve. Regardless of the initial amplitude of the free induction decay, the shape of the decay curve is always similar (Figure 39).

In normal soft tissues, T_1 is 150–2000 milliseconds, T_2 is 30–120 milliseconds, while T_2-star is 1–10 milliseconds. Comparing these relaxation times, we can see that T_2-star contributes the most to observed signal decay: The free induction decay signal falls to zero in 1–10 milliseconds. T_2 also contributes significantly, but the slight effect of T_1 can be ignored (Figure 40).

The decay of the signal after a single pulse — the free induction decay — is caused primarily by T_2 and T_2-star dephasing. It is T_2 that we wish to

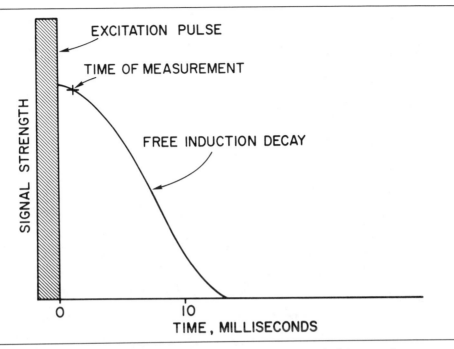

Figure 39. After a single excitation pulse, the sample re-emits a signal of the same frequency as the original excitation pulse. The signal is measured shortly after excitation, near its maximum, and falls to zero within a few milliseconds. This free induction decay signal contains the information for MRI image formation.

measure, but since its effect on the free induction decay is mixed with that of T_2-star, the free induction decay produced by single-pulse imaging cannot be used to measure T_2 alone. This is one of the motivations for developing pulse-sequencing. In the next section, we will see how it is possible, through the spin-echo pulse sequence, to use T_2-star to measure T_2. Another pulse sequence — inversion-recovery — can provide T_1 information.

Responses to Pulses of Varying Length

In the next experiment, we observe the effect of pulses of increasing duration on the amplitude of the re-emitted signal. Each pulse is followed by a signal which decays quickly but smoothly. We are not concerned with the shape of the decaying signal, but with its amplitude, which is maximal immediately following the pulse.

If we compared the initial amplitude of the signal following each pulse, we would see a striking effect. As we increase the pulse length starting from zero, the amplitude of the signal rises, becoming maximal at some particular pulse duration (here arbitrarily 10 microseconds). It then begins to decrease, falling to zero at 20 microseconds — twice the duration of the pulse producing the maximum. As the pulses are made still longer, another maximum is

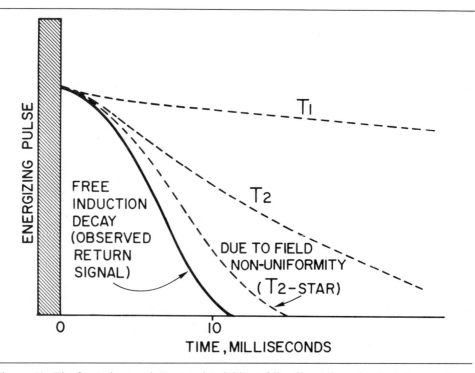

Figure 40. The free induction decay signal (solid line) falls off rapidly under the influence of three factors: energetic decay (T_1), dephasing due to thermal motion (T_2), and dephasing due to field nonuniformity (T_2-star). The dashed lines indicate the separate influence of each factor. T_2-star is the dominant source of signal loss.

found at 30 microseconds and another zero reading at 40 microseconds (Figure 41).

Why this peculiar relationship should exist between the length of the excitation pulse and the amplitude of the subsequent decaying signal is not immediately apparent.

In the last section we learned the relationship between the magnetization vector and signal strength. The magnetization vector expresses the response of all the magnetic nuclei in a voxel to stimulating radio pulses: A radio pulse drives the magnetization vector a certain number of degrees away from the positive Z-axis, depending on the strength of the pulse. Its projections on the longitudinal Z-axis and the transverse X-Y plane depend on the angle to which the magnetization vector is driven. The longitudinal component cannot be measured directly, but the transverse component is directly related to signal strength: The longer the transverse component, the stronger will be the received signal.

Although we might think that more energy applied to tissues would increase signal output, this is not the case: Only the transverse component of the magnetization vector induces a signal. The graph in Figure 41 represents

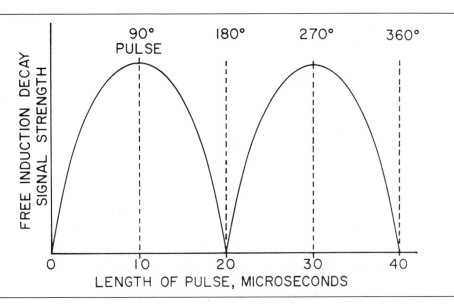

Figure 41. Exposing the sample to radio pulses of increasingly longer length results in remarkable changes in the amplitude of the free induction decay signal. Two maxima and three minima are observed: the maxima at 90° and 270° and the minima at zero, 180°, and 360°.

the change in length of the transverse component as the magnetization vector is rotated through 360°.

In this experiment, with this apparatus, the duration of the 90° pulse is actually determined by the sample size and transmitter power. Because a strong transmitter was used with a very small sample, the duration of the pulse needed to tip the magnetization vector of the sample was short — in the microsecond range. A weaker transmitter, or a larger sample, would require a pulse of longer duration to tip the magnetization vector 90° (Figure 42).

In clinical MRI scanners, the excitation transmitter can generate about 10,000 watts of power. Because the volume of tissue is very large, the duration of the 90° pulse might be 1–5 milliseconds. How much radio frequency power is needed to tip the vector 90° or 180° varies: The pulses must be tuned before each patient is examined, tailoring the pulse power to the volume of tissue to be excited.

PULSE SEQUENCING

MRI is magnetic interrogation of tissues: We ask a question of the tissues, listen to the body's answer, and analyze the response. The question we ask is in the form of radio-frequency energy, and the answer is in the form of the radio-frequency free induction decay signal picked up by the antenna. Coded into the signal is information about tissue properties. Understanding MRI image formation becomes a matter of understanding the relationships between the stimulating radio-frequency question and the tissue's answer.

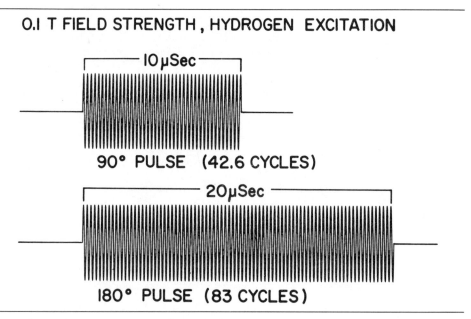

Figure 42. The strength of the pulse is determined by its length and intensity. In a given field strength, with a transmitter of fixed power output, a 180° pulse is twice as long as a 90° pulse.

In the last section we discussed, using the magnetization vector, the body's response to a single pulse, the simplest possible question; the smoothly-decaying signal from the tissues following the pulse is the simplest possible answer. The question this single pulse asks is, "What is the regional concentration of hydrogen?" The amplitude of the signal produced by a voxel of tissue would depend on its hydrogen content: An MRI scan based on a single pulse is largely a map of the distribution of hydrogen in the body and is of little diagnostic value.

However, almost all modern MRI asks more complex questions; usually, further tissue characterization is desired, including regional T_1 and T_2, and blood flow. These cannot be obtained using a single pulse; instead, pulse sequencing is used: A series of two or more radio pulses is applied to the tissues in quick succession. The use of a pulse sequence to stimulate the tissues results in a quite different type of signal from the tissues, containing information about tissue T_1 and T_2 characteristics, since the response to later pulses is influenced by earlier pulses in the sequence. A further elaboration of the pulse sequence can be made by repeating it after a lapse of time: The tissue is exposed to several rapid bursts of energy and, after a longer pause, to another series of rapid bursts. This repetition of the pulse sequence can provide still more tissue characterization. A specific pulse sequence is defined by the timing between individual pulses and between clusters of pulses.

Depending on the information we seek, the question asked by the pulse sequence must be phrased in a specific form. Factors affecting the formulation of the question include: (1) what region of the body is being examined and (2) what information is to be elicited (T_1, T_2, hydrogen distribution).

In formulating our questions, we are allowed several variables: (1) the strength of the individual pulses themselves (e.g., whether 90°, 180°, or other strengths), (2) the number of pulses in a sequence, (3) the time intervals between the pulses themselves (the interpulse interval, designated by the Greek letter tau), and (4) the time interval until the entire pulse sequence is repeated (the repetition time, TR). The interpulse interval is usually much shorter than time of repetition. These variables can be selected to elicit the desired information. The answers that the body gives to our different questions are in a special code contained in the signal from the tissues.

In the next section, we discuss the body's response to a specific pulse sequence — the spin-echo.

A COMMON PULSE SEQUENCE: SPIN ECHO

Having discussed tissue response to the simplest question — a single pulse of radio-frequency energy — we can explore tissue response to a more complicated question — the spin-echo pulse sequence. In the simplest form of this pulse sequence, the tissues are exposed to two pulses: a 90° pulse, followed some milliseconds later by a 180° pulse. In this example, the interpulse interval is 15 milliseconds.

As we would expect from the previous experiment, the response to the 90° pulse consists of a free-induction decay signal lasting a few milliseconds. By the time the 180° pulse is applied (15 milliseconds later), the signal is completely gone. As we would expect, the 180° pulse is not itself followed by a strong signal. However, an interesting phenomenon is observed some time after the 180° pulse: The sample re-radiates a signal which rises from zero to a distinct peak 15 milliseconds after the 180° pulse (and 30 milliseconds after the 90° pulse) (Figure 43).

Since this peak came at twice the time between the first and second pulses, it is referred to as an *echo* — by analogy to acoustic echo. It is actually an echo of the first (90°) free induction decay, made possible by the second (180°) pulse. It seemingly arises spontaneously, since it does not immediately follow a pulse. This separation from the relatively intense excitation pulse is an advantage because it allows the very weak return signal to be more clearly distinguished by the receiver.

If a person standing on an extended flat surface clapped his hands once, he would hear only the single sound directly from his hands. However, if there were a large vertical wall about 550 feet away, the person would hear, in addition to the actual clap, a second, weaker clap as an echo, about one second later. The sound (which travels at about 1100 feet per second) arrives at the barrier in one-half second, reverses its direction, and arrives back at its origin another one-half second later. The time of travel to the barrier was half the total time for echo return.

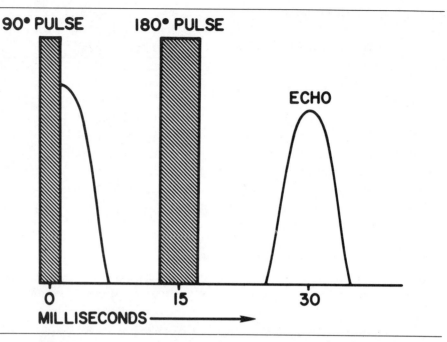

Figure 43. In a typical spin-echo pulse sequence, the sample is exposed to a 90° pulse, followed 15 milliseconds later by a 180° pulse. The 90° pulse is followed by free induction decay. Some time after the 180° pulse, a signal is emitted from the tissues, which rises to a peak at 30 milliseconds. The shape of this spin-echo is like two 90° free induction decay curves placed back-to-back.

The 180° magnetic pulse acts like a magnetic barrier in that it seems to cause an echo at twice the time interval between the 90° and 180° pulses. In MRI, this time-to-echo is abbreviated TE.

Origin of Spin-Echo

To understand why the echo is created after the 180° pulse, we need to briefly review why the free induction decay is destroyed after the 90° pulse.

The loss of the free induction decay signal is caused by dephasing. To review, in most tissues, T_1 is 150–2000 milliseconds, T_2 is approximately 30–120 milliseconds, and T_2-star is 1–10 milliseconds. In the 15 millisecond interpulse interval very little T_1 decay occurs, but substantial dephasing (due to T_2 and T_2-star) takes place, and the signal dies nearly completely before the second pulse.

Of the two sources of dephasing, the one that gives tissue characterization is thermal noise from the tissues themselves (T_2). The other (T_2-star), actually causes most of the free induction decay signal loss, but comes from fixed nonuniformity of the scanner's field. The two sources of dephasing are fundamentally different: T_2-star is constant (because it originates with constant nonuniformities) while T_2 fluctuates randomly (because it originates with thermal motion).

Dephasing Due to Constant Nonuniformity (T_2-star)

To understand the spin-echo phenomenon, consider first the effect of constant nonuniformities between different locations within the voxel under examination. Immediately after the 90° pulse, the phase coherence of all the nuclei in the voxel is high, the magnetization vector lies in the transverse plane rotating at the larmor frequency, and the free induction decay signal is maximal. If observed from a rotating frame, the magnetization vector would simply appear to lie stationary in the X–Y plane.

Mechanism of Echo

Due to T_2-star nonuniformities, the hydrogen nuclei at different locations within the voxel, which were originally locked in phase following the 90° pulse, precess at slightly higher or lower larmor frequencies and consequently lose their phase relationship. Because the nonuniformities are constant, the rates of precession of individual nuclei at various points in this field are constant, and the nuclei lose their phase coherence at a predictable rate.

The effect of the 180° pulse is to act as a magnetic barrier, making the nuclei come back into phase at the same rate as they went out of phase. As the nuclei come back into phase, the signals from the individual nuclei are again in phase, and a signal (the echo) is measured.

The reversal of the drifting apart of phase has been compared to a group of race horses that start simultaneously. Several seconds after they leave the starting gate, they occupy various positions along the track, because they are running at different speeds. If their direction were somehow instantaneously reversed, and they continued to run at the same speeds, they would, after a period of time equal to that between the start and the reversal, arrive back at the gate simultaneously.

The 90° pulse is analogous to the release from the gate. The 180° pulse is the unnamed mechanism for causing the horses to change direction; their arrival back at the starting gate is the spin echo. Because it takes as long to come back into phase (after the 180° pulse) as it took to go out of phase, the time-to-echo is twice the 90°–180° pulse interval.

To analyze this dephasing and refocusing in terms of the magnetization vector (from a rotating frame of reference): As the nuclei dephased after the initial excitation pulse, the magnetization vector would appear to lie in the transverse plane and to break into many smaller vectors, drifting clockwise and counterclockwise at constant rates, like a fan being opened. The 180° pulse would cause the motion of these vectors to reverse. Subsequently, at the time of echo, we would see the many smaller vectors come back together, like a fan being closed. (A more detailed explanation of spin-echo using the magnetization vector is to be found in Figures 44 and 45.)

The spin-echo produced by the 180° pulse is actually an echo of the free induction decay. The echo can be considered a resurrection and doubling of

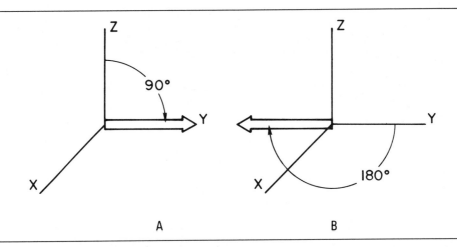

Figure 44. A 90° pulse drives the magnetization vector into the transverse plane (A). A 180° pulse applied immediately after the 90° pulse rotates the vector into the opposite side of the transverse plane (B). If there is no time interval between the two pulses, they are equivalent to a single 270° pulse and produce a free induction decay signal. If, instead, a short interval of time is allowed between the 90° and 180° pulses, the phenomenon of spin-echo occurs.

the apparently vanished 90° free induction decay. Its shape is determined by the free induction decay curve: Because the nuclei come into phase at the same rate as they went out of phase, the echo curve is symmetrical; the rising half of the echo curve is the mirror image of the free induction decay curve. After reaching maximum coherence, the nuclei again go out of phase at approximately the same rate as after the initial 90° pulse: The falling half of the echo curve very closely reproduces the original free induction decay curve.

It is possible, by repeating several 180° pulses at appropriate intervals, to produce several echoes after the initial 90° pulse. Each new 180° pulse has the effect of reversing the constant dephasing that has occurred since the previous pulse. The ability of pulse sequencing to produce multiple spin-echoes demonstrates the indestructibility of T_2-star dephasing, since echoes can be resurrected several times by subsequent 180° pulses, following a single 90° pulse (Figure 46).

From this discussion, we see that the spin echo is an artifact due to inherent, fixed T_2-star non uniformity of the MRI scanner's main field, gradient fields, and nonuniformity of tissue magnetic susceptibility. In itself the echo has nothing to do with tissue T_2. *If, somehow, these constant nonuniformities could be eliminated and the field could be made perfectly uniform, no spin-echo would occur.*

T_2 from Spin-echo

The constancy of the field nonuniformities throughout the voxel being imaged causes T_2-star dephasing to occur at a constant rate. The effect of the

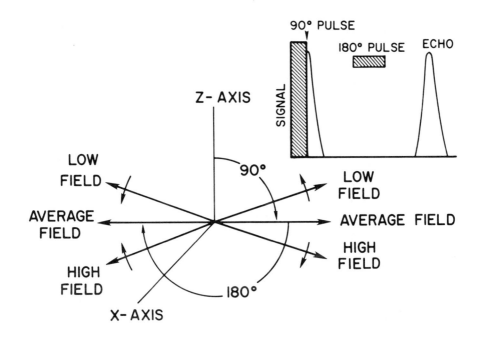

Figure 45. In the short interval of time between the 90° and 180° pulses, some dephasing of nuclei occurs. The direction of phase shift is indicated by the arrows on the vectors fanning out clockwise and counterclockwise in the transverse plane, to the right of the Z-axis.

After the 180° pulse, they lie in the opposite side of the transverse plane (to the left of the Z-axis). The arrows on these vectors indicate that the nuclei are coming back into phase.

As the nuclei go out of phase (after the 90° pulse) the signal falls off. As they come back into phase (some time after the 180° pulse) the echo signal is produced. The phenomenon of spin–echo occurs because dephasing and rephasing occur at constant rates, due to T_2-star constant nonuniformities of field strength.

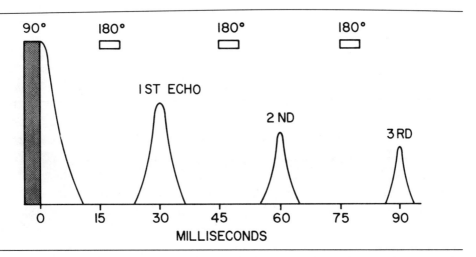

Figure 46. By repeating 180° pulses after the initial 90° pulse, multiple echoes can be generated.

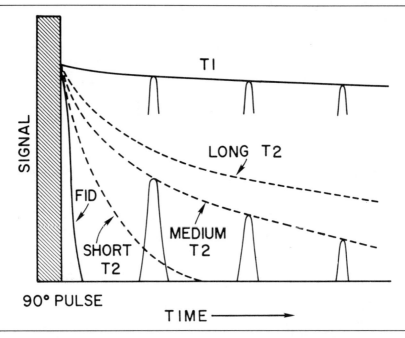

Figure 47. If the only source of dephasing were T_2-star constant nonuniformities of field, the only source of echo degradation would be T_1 (energy loss). This hypothetical case is shown at top by the solid line connecting tips of echoes.

But in tissues, repeated echoes decline much more rapidly due to T_2 (random, thermal motion dephasing). Dashed lines indicate erosion of multiple echoes in tissues with short, medium, and long T_2.

180° pulse is to cause the nuclei to come back into phase at the same rate as they went out of phase.

While the dephasing effects of T_2-star can be reversed by a 180° pulse, those of T_2, cannot, due to their random nature. The echo is thus weaker than the free induction decay by the amount of T_2 dephasing that has occurred during the time to echo.

T_2-star creates the echo, T_2 erodes it.

T_2 represents unpredictable dephasing which nibbles away at the spin echo. In multiple-echo sequences, the height of successive echoes decreases by T_2. If regional numerical measurements of T_2 are sought, they can be calculated from the rate of erosion between two or more successive echoes from the region (Figure 47).

T_2 has a significant effect on the echo, because in most T_2-weighted sequences the time to echo is chosen to span the likely T_2 values of the tissues. Most healthy tissue has a T_2 in the range of 20–100 milliseconds; the time to echo is made to fall in the range of 30–120 milliseconds.

In clinical MRI, scans usually are constructed from the spin–echo, rather than from the free induction decay following the 90° pulse. In a common spin-echo sequence, three stimulating pulses are used: the 90° pulse, followed at 15 and 45 milliseconds by 180° pulses, giving rise to two echoes, at 30 and

60 milliseconds. In regions of short T_2, rapid degradation of the echo occurs, the signal measured is weaker, and the region appears darker. Similarly, in regions of long T_2, less degradation occurs, the signal is stronger, and the region remains bright.

Where there is a region of interest with a long T_2, this can be emphasized by using longer interpulse intervals to produce later echoes. By the time of the later pulses, the regions of short T_2 have eroded their regional echoes and appear dark, while regions of long T_2 are correspondingly associated with a strong echo signal and appear bright against the surrounding healthy brain. For example, by delaying the 180° pulses (e.g., to 45 or 60 milliseconds after the 90° pulse), later spin echoes (e.g., at 90 or 120 milliseconds) are obtained, and these are useful in detecting regions with pathologically prolonged T_2. By 120 milliseconds, the signal will have disappeared from most healthy tissues, except cerebrospinal fluid (which has a much longer T_2), and the brain itself will appear dark. A pathological region of long T_2 could still be producing an echo at this time and would appear bright.

Gradient Echoes

It is possible to use gradient magnetic fields in place of 180° radio-frequency pulses to cause the reversal of phasing that produces the echo. A constant gradient in the Z-axis is applied following the 90° pulse. This now dominates other fixed field nonuniformities to establish the direction of phase drift. At the time a 180° pulse would normally be applied, the polarity of the gradient is reversed, but its strength is exactly the same as before reversal. This reversed gradient causes the phase drift of the nuclei to reverse and refocus, thereby creating an echo. An advantage of using gradients to produce echoes is that exposure of the tissue to the substantial amount of radio-frequency energy in the 180° pulses is avoided. Heating of tissue is less of a problem.

T_1 from Spin-Echo

In spin echo pulse sequencing, T_2 had a significant effect on the strength of the spin-echo signal, because for most tissues the time-to-echo is made comparable to T_2 of tissues. On the other hand, T_1 has little effect on the spin echo because it is much longer than the time-to-echo. In the examples above, the time-to-echo of the last echo was 120 milliseconds; T_1 of most tissues is 150–2000 milliseconds. How is it possible to encode T_1 information into the scan?

In practice, the tissues are not simply exposed to a single spin-echo pulse sequence of one 90° pulse, followed by one or more 180° pulses. Instead, the spin-echo pulse sequence is repeated at intervals of 0.5–5.0 seconds. This interval is called the *repetition time*, abbreviated TR. For example, at a repetition time of 0.5 seconds, a 90° pulse is applied to the tissues every 0.5 seconds. Using the same interpulse interval as before, each 90° pulse is followed 15 milliseconds later by a 180° pulse (Figure 48).

As we would expect, each 90° pulse is immediately followed by a free-

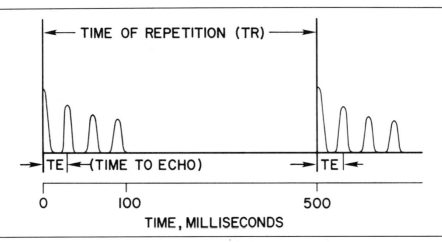

Figure 48. The most common pulse sequencing used in MRI consists of repeated multiple spin-echo sequences, separated by repetition time TR. In this example TR is 500 milliseconds. The length of the repetition time affects the amplitude of the next free induction decay, resulting in T_1 weighting. How changing repetition time affects the free induction decay of the next 90° pulse is shown in Figure 49.

induction decay signal and, 30 milliseconds later, by an echo signal. During these 30 milliseconds, the echo will be degraded at a rate T_2.

When the repetition time is made comparable to the T_1's of various tissues, the size of the free induction decay (and thus the spin-echo) in the repeated pulse sequences are different for different tissues; T_1 information is encoded into the scan: The scan becomes T_1-weighted.

To understand why the initial pulse-sequence can affect subsequent pulse sequences, we need to review T_1 energy loss: A voxel of tissue absorbs a certain amount of energy from a 90° pulse; it loses this energy at rate T_1. This loss of energy is unrelated to the dephasing and rephasing (from T_2 and T_2-star), which occur at a much faster rate and which cause the short free induction decay.

The energy loss starts immediately after the initial 90° pulse and continues long after the last echo, because T_1 is so much larger than T_2 and T_2-star. Although the tissue is silent after the last spin-echo signal, this does not mean that the nuclei in the tissue have returned to their equilibrium state; they still possess energy, which they continue to lose.

Dephasing and energy loss can be visualized using the longitudinal and transverse components of the magnetization vector. While the transverse component is dephasing and rephasing, producing the free induction decay and echo signals, the longitudinal component is growing in the positive Z-direction at the much slower rate T_1. When the transverse component has completely dephased (and shrunk to zero) after the spin-echo, the longitudinal component has regained only a fraction of its original (prestimulation) length; it continues to grow at rate T_1.

If the next repetition of the pulse sequence is started at a time comparable to T_1 of a region, its 90° pulse encounters a region of tissue still partially

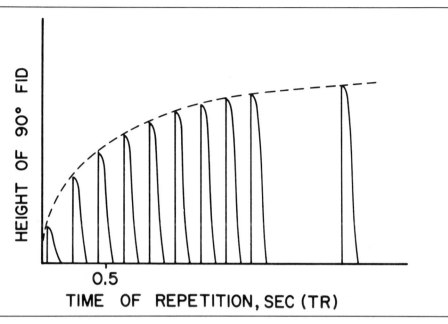

Figure 49. This figure shows the amplitude of the free induction decay of a repeated pulse sequence and its relationship to repetition time. At short repetition times, the region has little time to undergo T_1 relaxation and cannot absorb much energy from the next 90° pulse; its free induction decay is correspondingly small. At longer repetition times, the region has more time to undergo T_1 relaxation, absorbs more energy from the pulse, and its free induction decay is stronger.

energized (whose longitudinal component has not regained its original length). The result of this is that the tissue cannot absorb all of the energy that it might from the new 90° pulse. The subsequent free induction decay and its spin-echo in the new pulse sequence are correspondingly weaker. On scans constructed from the echo signals of the new pulse sequence, the region appears darker.

In our earlier discussion, we saw that the voxels in a plane of tissue, when exposed to a single 90° pulse, give free induction decays of comparable amplitude because of their similar water content. In repeated pulse sequences, the amount of energy a voxel absorbs from a 90° pulse (and the strength of its free induction decay) will depend on how much energy has been lost from the voxel by the time of the next 90° pulse. *Because the echo for each voxel is a resurrection of its free induction decay, the heights of the spin echoes for the voxels will also reflect T_1.*

In general, for a given tissue voxel, the amplitude of its free induction decay increases with more prolonged repetition time, because the tissues have more time to undergo T_1 relaxation and are able to absorb more energy from the new pulse (Figure 49).

Using short and long repetition times, we will see how the scans they produce are correspondingly T_1- and T_2-weighted.

The first repetition time to be examined is 0.5 seconds. This repetition time is effective in creating T_1 contrast of tissues, because T_1's of various tissues are scattered above and below 0.5 seconds. At 0.5 seconds after the initial 90° pulse, regions of long T_1 still retain much of their energy, while regions of short T_1 have almost completely relaxed. Because these regions differ in their degree of energy retention, they absorb differing amounts of energy from the new 90° pulse. Regions with long T_1 will have decayed less and will absorb less energy from the next 90° pulse; their subsequent free induction decay and echoes will be correspondingly weaker. Regions with short T_1 have, by 0.5 seconds, lost most of their energy; they absorb more energy from the second 90° pulse and have a larger free induction decay (and echo) after the second 90° pulse. When MRI scans are reconstructed from echoes of the repeated pulse sequence, these images show regions of long T_1 as darker than those of short T_1.

Fat, for example, which has a T_1 of about 150 milliseconds, goes through about three T_1's by 0.5 seconds and will appear bright on the image. A tissue with a very long T_1, such as cerebrospinal fluid, hardly relaxes at all before the second pulse and will still appear dark (Figure 50).

At a repetition time of about 0.5 seconds, MRI scans are "T_1-weighted," meaning that the brightness of various tissues reflects their T_1.

If the repetition time is extended to 2.0 seconds, longer than the T_1 of most cellular tissues, this is enough time for the tissues in the slice being imaged to lose their energy and return to their prestimulation state. Each succeeding pulse sequence encounters tissues that are all essentially in an unstimulated state; T_1 has little effect on the free induction decay or echoes of the successive pulse sequences. Most regions produce, after the new 90° pulse, free induction decays that are large and comparable in amplitude, because hydrogen content of various soft tissues is fairly uniform. Apparent T_1 regional differences are minimal and T_1 does not affect contrast on the final scan.

The exception to this range of T_1's is cerebrospinal fluid, which has a T_1 close to that of pure water (about 2.7 seconds). It still retains a substantial amount of energy at 2.0 seconds, when the next pulse sequence starts; it absorbs less energy from the next 90° pulse and appears relatively dark on the image against the brighter cellular tissues.

With long repetition times, the free-induction decay signals produced from various cellular tissues are all strong and equal, but the efficiency with which the echoes are produced varies from region to region, as a function of regional T_2. Regions of long T_2 appear brighter, while those of short T_2 appear darker. MRI scans made from the spin echoes of a 2.0 second repetition time reflect almost entirely regional T_2 and are T_2-weighted.

By using repetition times of between 0.5 and 2.0 seconds, MRI scans can present a combination of T_1- and T_2-weighting, the proportion of T_1 versus T_2 weighting depending on the repetition time. Longer repetition times minimize regional differences in T_1, thus allowing T_2 to dominate regional image brightness. Repetition times of 4–5 seconds and a time-to-echo of perhaps 200 milliseconds produce a bright cerebrospinal fluid with almost no

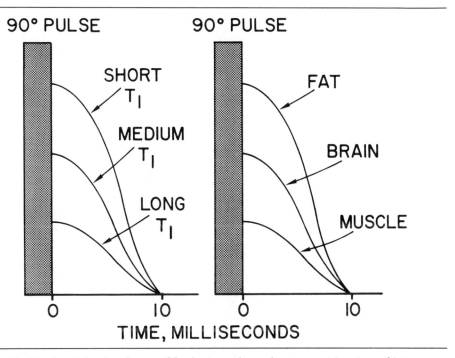

Figure 50. The free induction decays of fat, brain, and muscle at a repetition time of 0.5 seconds. A tissue with a short T_1 (such as fat) will have undergone nearly complete T_1 relaxation; consequently it absorbs more energy, has a large free induction decay curve, and appears bright. Brain, with a medium-long T_1, undergoes less relaxation and has a smaller free induction decay curve. Muscle, with its long T_1, undergoes the least relaxation, gives the weakest free induction decay curve and appears dark.

visible soft tissue. It appears like an old-fashioned myelogram, with iodinated oil replacing spinal fluid.

SOURCES OF REGIONAL IMAGE BRIGHTNESS

An MRI scan displays a slice of tissue as regions of varying brightness. Each scan has on it a line of print stating the repetition time and time-to-echo. Clinical images are usually created using repeated spin–echo pulse sequences; the image is formed from the echoes. The brightness of a region in the image depends upon the strength (amplitude) of its spin–echo signal. To understand regional brightness and its relation to tissue characterization, it may be helpful to summarize the factors determining this echo strength.

There are two factors influencing the amplitude of the spin echo: the height of the free induction decay (of which the echo is the resurrection) and the amount of T_2 decay that occurs between the free induction decay and echo.

When the free induction decay signal is stronger, the echo signal following it will be correspondingly stronger. From the above discussion, we know that the free induction decay of successive pulse sequences is a function of the relation between the region's T_1 and the length of the repetition time, which separates the repeated pulse sequences. At long repetition times (of 2.0 or

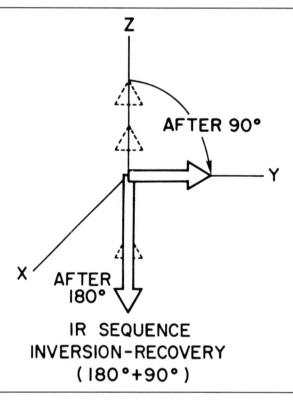

Z

AFTER 90°

Y

X

AFTER
180°

IR SEQUENCE
INVERSION-RECOVERY
(180°+90°)

Figure 51. The inversion-recovery pulse sequence consists of a 180° pulse followed some time later by a 90° pulse. After the 180° pulse, the longitudinal component grows in the positive Z direction at rate T_1. The 90° pulse tilts the vector into the transverse plane, providing a measurable signal.

more seconds) the effect of T_1 on the free induction decay is minimal, and all voxels in a plane of tissue produce free induction decays of comparable amplitude. At these long repetition times, T_1 contrast is removed. With shorter repetition times, comparable to T_1 of tissues, the heights of the free induction decays of different voxels become differentiated according to their T_1. A repetition time of 0.5 seconds tends to emphasize T_1 of soft tissues: The scan is T_1-weighted.

Whatever the height of the free induction decay, its echo signals will be degraded at the rate T_2; some T_2 information is always included in the scan. Scans made with a repetition time of 0.5 seconds, although T_1-weighted, still contain T_2 information. With longer repetition times (of 2.0 seconds, for instance) T_1 information is minimized, leaving the dephasing effects of T_2 as the primary source of differences in echo strength between different regions: the scan is T_2-weighted.

INVERSION-RECOVERY

Another pulse sequence commonly in clinical use is the inversion-recovery pulse sequence. This sequence has the advantage of measuring T_1 and almost

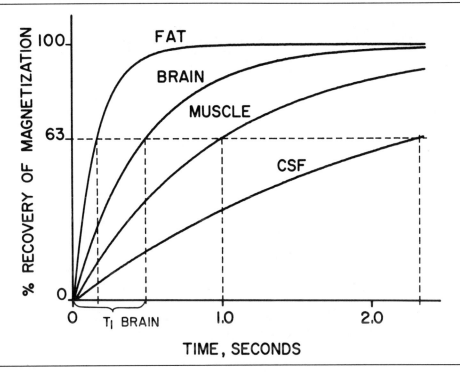

Figure 52. Fat, brain, muscle, and CSF are shown undergoing T_1 relaxation after a 180° pulse. Each tissue is recovering at a different rate: At 0.5 seconds the three cellular tissues are widely separated in their percentage of recovery; an inversion-recovery scan made at this pulse separation shows considerable contrast between these four tissues.

At two seconds, the three cellular tissues have nearly completely relaxed; the CSF requires substantially longer. A scan made with this pulse separation shows little contrast among the cellular tissues, but strong CSF/cellular tissue contrast.

eliminating T_2 effects from the scan. It provides finer anatomical detail and better gray-white matter contrast than T_2-weighted scans.

In inversion-recovery, a 180° pulse is applied to the tissues first, followed by a 90° pulse after an interval of time comparable to T_1 of the tissues (in the following example, 0.5 seconds). The 180° pulse inverts the magnetization vector from the positive Z-axis to the negative Z-axis. Because the magnetization vector is entirely longitudinal, there is no transverse component and no emitted signal. Immediately after excitation, the magnetization vector begins to grow in the positive Z-direction at rate T_1. How much the vector grows in the positive Z-direction during 0.5 seconds is directly related to the T_1 of tissue in the voxel, but cannot be measured.

To create a measurable transverse component, a 90° pulse is applied to the tissues. This pulse tips the longitudinal magnetization vector into the transverse plane, and a free induction decay signal follows the pulse. The strength of the free induction decay will be related to the amount of T_1 decay that has occurred since the initial 180° pulse (Figures 51 and 52).

This free induction decay signal may be measured directly, or, because it is

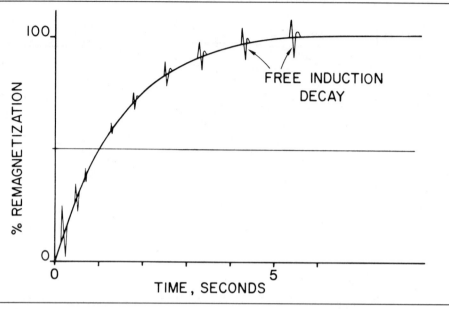

Figure 53. The solid rising curve represents T_1 recovery after the initial 180° pulse. The spikes represent the free induction decay following the 90° pulse after the indicated pulse separation. The amplitude of the free induction decay signal is the same at two different times after the initial 180° pulse. From a scan made with a specific pulse separation, it is impossible to determine what degree of relaxation the tissue has undergone (compare to Figure 33).

difficult to measure the re-emitted signal directly after the intense burst of energy in the 90° pulse, an early echo of the free induction decay can be produced by applying a 180° pulse soon (perhaps 10 milliseconds) after the 90° pulse, producing an echo (at 20 milliseconds) as in the standard spin–echo sequence. Using the echo in this way to measure the free-induction decay indirectly introduces some slight T_2 effect into the scan.

One problem with the inversion recovery pulse sequence is the lack of a simple relationship between T_1 and the amplitude of the free-induction decay signal, and thus regional image brightness (Figure 53).

OTHER PULSE SEQUENCES

The spin-echo pulse sequences described in this chapter are the most common in clinical use. Many others have been developed, but cannot be covered here. However, most of the principles involved are the same.

It is widely believed (and probably correctly) that much of the future development of MRI will be in the development of new pulse sequences. Great potential exists in this area, because there are many variables that can be used in designing a pulse sequence. Some of these were mentioned earlier in this chapter: pulse strength, the number of pulses, and the temporal separation of the pulses. Although not covered in depth here, there are several other possible variables: the intensity, direction, and timing of gradients; and the phase distortion of the signal from different regions of the image.

Each of these factors influences, in some way, the signal elicited from the tissues. Each pulse sequence is a strategy that asks a specific question of the tissues; the answer to each question is encoded in the free induction decay signal. The signal measured is very complex and must be analyzed by the scanner's computer for a useable image to be reconstructed. The computer software controlling the execution of the pulse sequence and the reconstruction of the final image can be regarded as another variable.

CHAPTER 6: THE MRI SCANNER

A clinical MRI scanner superficially resembles a CT scanner: There is a large gantry into which the patient is placed, a complex of computers, a control console, and various pieces of electronic apparatus. However, the dimensions of the gantries are quite different.

In most MRI systems, the space into which the patient is placed is much longer than in a CT scanner: It is a cylinder about two meters long; its diameter is one half to one third its length. This size and shape is important in patient management, in that the anatomical region to be examined must occupy the center of this cylindrical volume, so the patient must be fully inside the gantry.

The dimensions of the gantry are dictated by the size and placement of the several coils needed to generate the various magnetic fields used in MRI imaging. The magnetic fields produced are roughly analogous to the Earth's magnetic field in our earlier compass analogy. In our discussion of imaging (Chapter 3), we saw how localization is achieved by means of the magnetic gradient, a magnetic field which changes strength gradually between one position in space and another: The resonant larmor frequency of a hydrogen nucleus depends on its position in the gradient. An analogous magnetic gradient is the one in the Earth's field, which could be used to localize a compass needle on the Earth's surface.

In MRI, magnetic gradients are produced using the principle of superimposition: When a volume of space is exposed to several different magnetic fields, the resultant field is the sum of the individual fields. The magnetic field required for MRI must be very strong, but in order to form the required gradient, it need vary in strength only slightly from one edge of the imaged volume to the other. The gradient field in MRI scanners consists of weak gradient magnetic fields superimposed on a strong, uniform field (the main field).

The strength of the main field is the most common characteristic used to describe a scanner: Current clinical scanners range in strength from 0.02 to 2.0 tesla. (One tesla is 10,000 gauss.) In addition to being extremely strong, the main field must also be extremely uniform spatially. Throughout the scan time, this field remains constant. Onto the main, uniform field are superimposed the weaker, nonuniform gradient fields, which typically increase in strength by about one gauss per centimeter through the region being imaged. This represents a change in main field strength of about 0.25% from one edge of the cross section to the other.

The main field is on continuously throughout the course of an MRI scan, but the gradient fields switch on and off and change intensities many times. The main field and gradient fields are generated by different sets of coils within the scanner gantry (except permanent magnet scanners, which do not use coils to generate the main field). In terms of cost, those producing the main field are most important.

MAIN FIELD MAGNETS

In most clinical MRI scanners now marketed, the main field is generated by electromagnets, either superconductive or resistive. A third type of magnet, the permanent magnet, is marketed by only one major company, but shows promise for future development. The type of magnet is often used to classify the entire scanner: it is either a *resistive, superconductive,* or *permanent magnet* scanner.

Until recently, it was thought that the method of creating the main field was of paramount importance in establishing the quality of a scanner. But with experience it has become clear that there is much more to a scanner than the main field and that gradient and antenna coil design, excitation and reception coils, computer software, and scanning strategies (pulse sequencing) are each critical elements in the system, and that each is but a link in a chain of quality. This does not diminish the importance of the main field quality, but to classify (and thus judge) the entire scanner on the basis of the main field's strength and the means of generating it is unjustifiable.

ELECTROMAGNETS

Both resistive and superconductive electromagnets are based on a principle demonstrated by Danish scientist Hans Christian Ørsted early in the nineteenth century: When an electric current passes through a wire, a magnetic field is created about the wire. The strength of this field diminishes with the

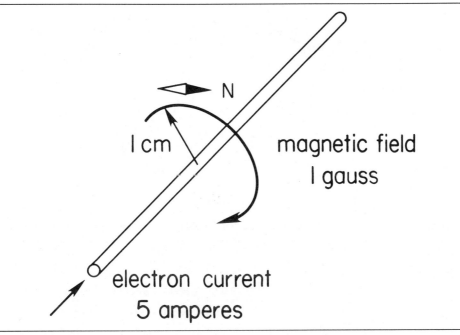

N

I cm

magnetic field
I gauss

electron current
5 amperes

Figure 54. Current passing through a wire creates a magnetic field around the wire. The direction of the field follows the right-hand rule: if one extends the thumb of the right hand in the direction of the current, the magnetic field is the direction of the four curled fingers, indicated by the direction of the compass. By definition, the strength of the magnetic field one centimeter from a wire carrying five amperes of current is one gauss.

distance from the wire (see Figure 54). The principle of electromagnetism has been used in many electronic devices, but using electromagnets to create the large volume of uniform field required by clinical MRI has been an engineering challenge.

The details of electromagnet construction vary from design to design, but in general several circular coils encircle the region of the body to be examined. The coils are housed in the gantry of the scanner, and each coil is made of many strands of wire or metal foil. The coils are precisely shaped and positioned and the electron current passing through them is constant. The size of the coils and the geometry of their placement allows the creation of an acceptably uniform field through the volume of tissue being imaged; the constancy of the electric current ensures the stability of the magnetic field during the time needed for imaging.

To understand the approach taken to create a uniform field by electromagnets, we can note a theoretical model developed in the nineteenth century: If an infinitely fine wire were spirally wound around the surface of a non-magnetic sphere and an electric current passed through the wire, the magnetic field created in the cavity of the sphere would be perfectly uniform (Figure 55). Such a magnet is not used, for practical reasons: This design

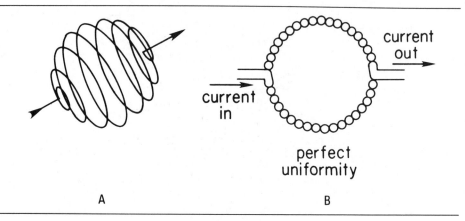

current
out

current
in

perfect
uniformity

A   B

Figure 55. In a theoretical model, current passed through a fine wire wound spirally around an imaginary sphere produces a uniform field within the sphere, shown (A) obliquely and (B) in midline cross section.

leaves no access holes for the patient; the creation of access holes would cause the field to bulge out of these holes, distorting the field. Although it is not used in practice, knowledge of this theoretical model allows us to understand the designs used in resistive and superconductive systems, both of which use circular coils of conductor to achieve uniformity of field.

The major problem to overcome in the design of electromagnets is electrical resistance. At room temperature, every metal exhibits electrical resistance, producing heat when an electric current is passed through it. The manner in which this electrical resistance is dealt with defines the two types of electromagnets. In resistive MRI scanners, the wire is allowed to stay near room temperature and the heat produced is physically removed. In superconductive MRI scanners, the wire is cooled to temperatures near absolute zero, at which the metal loses its resistance, and the electric current flows without producing heat.

RESISTIVE SCANNERS: GEOMETRY OF COIL ARRANGEMENT

In resistive scanners, four coils are used to produce the main magnetic field. They are parallel to one another and the outer two are smaller in diameter than the inner two, so that the four coils approximate the surface of a sphere, like parallels of latitude on a globe. Although this design does not produce perfect uniformity in the entire volume contained by the coils, it does create acceptable uniformity in a large enough volume to be useful for imaging (Figure 56).

The four coil arrangement approximates a sphere; but the end coils are made smaller than the surface of a sphere to create a slightly higher field near these apertures, thus tending to repel the bulging field back inside to compensate for the defect in magnetic field produced by the patient access holes.

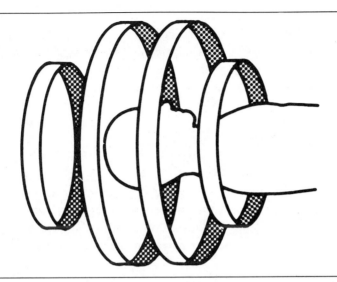

Figure 56. In resistive scanners, four separate coils of a size and position which approximate a sphere are used. This permits patient access, while providing acceptible uniformity in a sufficiently large volume.

In resistive scanners the coils are made of either foils or wire of a highly conductive metal, such as copper or aluminum. The two main manufacturers of resistive magnets use aluminum foil strips (about 15 centimeters wide) wound spirally in several thousand layers in each coil.

Heat Production

Although aluminum is a good conductor of electrons, it does offer measurable resistance and consequent heat production. Copper is a 40% better conductor, but aluminum is favored because of its lower cost and weight. Aluminum is less than one third as dense as copper but produces about half again as much heat.

The use of aluminum as a conductor limits field strength to about 1500 gauss (0.15 tesla). This limitation is due to the heat dissipated in the aluminum by the very large electric currents required. To create a 1500 gauss field requires 200–250 amperes of electric current, which in an MRI resistive coil system generates about 50 kilowatts of heat. To double the field strength would require doubling the electric current, which, unfortunately, results in quadrupling the heat dissipation. To raise the field strength to 3000 gauss would dissipate 200 kilowatts of heat. Fifty kilowatts is manageable, but supplying and removing 200 kilowatts of heat in a hospital setting would be prohibitive.

Heat from the aluminum foil is dissipated by passing deionized water past each coil assembly and on to an external heat-exchanger. This 50 kilowatts of heat is approximately the amount produced by a passenger automobile engine; the heat exchanger is equivalent to the automobile's radiator.

A further problem in generating a magnetic field using resistive magnets is the production of strong continuous electric current. Any fluctuation in the electric current results in a corresponding fluctuation of the magnetic field. Power supplies capable of regulating the current to one part in a million are available at a reasonable cost. The field is correspondingly constant over time.

Field uniformity in resistives

Field uniformity is poorer with resistive magnets than with superconductive magnets for several reasons. First, the volume of uniformity is smaller. In general, the larger the magnet relative to the patient, the greater will be the volume of acceptable uniformity. In resistive magnets, the coils are made small, to reduce the amount of aluminum used in the coil, in an attempt to minimize heat production. This small coil size constricts the size of the volume of high uniformity.

No resistive coils are perfectly shaped, nor are they perfectly spaced. The four independent coil units in the usual resistive system are difficult to position and maintain exactly parallel and undistorted when the current is turned on to create the main field. The main field produces magnetomotive forces which tend to pull the coils toward their common center.

As with superconductive systems, ferromagnetic materials (structural steel, etc.) in the external environment of the magnet further distort the external field and thus the field within the magnet. Shimming can be used to fine tune the magnet and counteract such distortion. To this end, movable ferrous rods can be positioned outside the coils. In resistive systems, threaded adjustments are often provided to position the coils. Variable electromagnetic coils can also be used for shimming.

The electron current supply is very stable but, inevitably, imperfectly regulated. As a consequence, the magnetic field necessarily fluctuates slightly.

Despite their limited field strength, resistive main coils have some attractive features: Manufacturing cost is low compared to superconductive coils, electrical power cost is only six to ten dollars per hour while operating, and they can easily be turned off when not in use. Even at the low field strengths of most resistive systems (0.02–0.2 tesla), good clinical images are produced. Resistive scanners cannot, however, meet the field strength and uniformity requirements for some applications, such as chemical shift spectroscopy.

SUPERCONDUCTIVE MAGNETS

Most metals show an electrical resistance which is roughly proportional to their absolute temperature (measured in degrees Kelvin). Cooling causes their resistance to drop. The resistance of the tungsten filament in an incandescent light bulb at room temperature, when the bulb is unlit, is only about one tenth that when it is lit, and the filament heated.

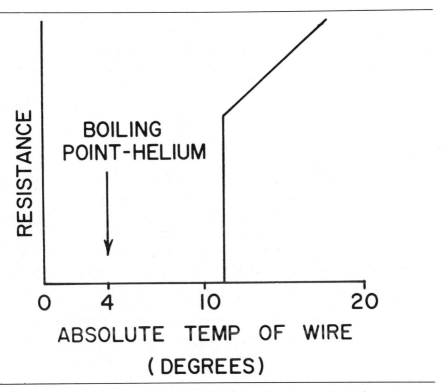

Figure 57. When cooled, most metals show a drop in electrical resistance. Some show a complete loss of resistance (superconductivity) near absolute zero.

The resistance of most metals shows a nearly linear drop as they are cooled to absolute zero from higher temperatures. With many metals, at a specific critical temperature a few degrees above absolute zero, the resistance falls abruptly to zero (Figure 57); their conductivity becomes infinite and they are said to be superconductive. An electric current started in a superconductive wire circulates indefinitely.

The temperature at which superconductivity occurs varies from metal to metal and alloy to alloy. Ordinary lead (Pb), for instance, becomes superconductive below 7.4° Kelvin. In MRI, it is desirable to use conducting metals whose critical temperatures are as high as possible. The niobium–titanium alloys used in MRI scanners become superconductive at temperatures in the range of 10–20° Kelvin. The coils are cooled by liquid helium, which boils at 4.2° Kelvin.

In 1987, a new class of ceramic superconductors was announced. They are superconducting temperature greater than 100° Kelvin, allowing cooling with only liquid nitrogen. If these materials can be fabricated into dependable wires, much less expensive MRI superconductive magnets may be possible.

At installation, the coils of the MRI scanner are cooled, the current is started and, when the desired field strength is reached, a superconductive link is closed. No further power is required. For practical purposes, the current runs indefinitely (so long as adequate cooling is maintained), and only a few gauss drop in field strength occurs each year. Because the flow of electric current is constant, the magnetic field created within the MRI scanner is constant; it is essentially a permanent magnet.

Coil Configuration

In resistive systems, conductor length is minimized in order to reduce heat dissipation. Because there is no electrical resistance in superconductive magnets, no heat is produced, and there is no longer a critical constraint on the length of wire used, so more coils of a larger diameter can be used; coil diameters as large as two meters have been manufactured. As the coils become large relative to the patient, the uniformity within the volume being imaged becomes greater.

In resistive magnets, we saw how four coils conforming to the surface of a sphere were used to create a uniform magnetic field. The coils of a superconductive magnet are constructed on a precision-machined cylinder (usually aluminum) and so have the same diameter. On its outer surface are grooves for the coils of niobium-titanium conductor. The conductors are clustered in groups of four or six, with the higher number of turns near the ends of the cylinder. Although the coils have the same diameter, placing more turns of conductor at the ends of the cylinder than near its center minimizes bulging of the field at the openings; an effect comparable to that of the hypothetical wrapped sphere is created (Figure 58).

The cylinder and its coils are suspended in liquid helium. The helium container is suspended in a vacuum chamber which, in turn, is surrounded by liquid nitrogen (70° Kelvin) and this in turn is surrounded by an evacuated chamber. This rather elaborate assembly is understandably expensive and requires considerable expertise in order to make a reliable product. Two commercial firms make essentially all of the clinical superconductive magnets at present.

Liquid Gas

Liquid nitrogen is readily available, but liquid helium is not. The cost of the latter is correspondingly variable. It is present in underground natural gas deposits due to alpha decay of long-lived radioactive substances such as thorium and its daughters. Because it is a noble monatomic gas and has an atomic mass of only four, helium has a low boiling point, making it easily isolated from natural gas by liquefaction. Since helium cannot burn, it is a useless component if it remains with the gas. Although easily produced by anyone having a substantial supply of natural gas, there has not been wide-

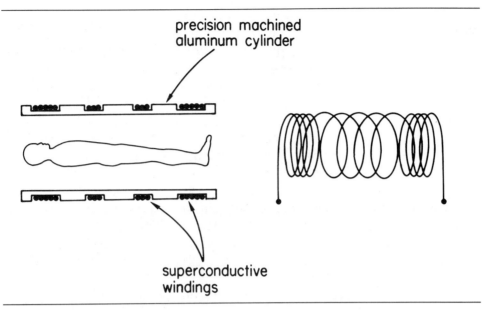

precision machined
aluminum cylinder

superconductive
windings

Figure 58. In superconductive MRI scanners, the coils are positioned in grooves on the outside of a precision-machined cylinder of aluminum. Acceptable field uniformity is obtained by using more turns of wire near the ends of the cylinder.

spread recovery of helium (and particularly its liquefaction) because of the lack of a commercial market.

Preventing helium boil-off from the scanner is a formidable problem and can best be appreciated by thinking of the outside room as an oven some 300° Celsius hotter than the liquid helium. Typically, loss of helium from a superconductive magnet is about 500 milliliters per hour, vented to the outside atmosphere. At the 1987 liquid helium price of about five dollars per liter, annual helium cost is $15,000–20,000. Added to this is the cost of liquid nitrogen. Although a greater volume of this boils off than of helium, it is very much less expensive. If helium loss is considered a serious economic problem, closed refrigeration systems are available to reliquify the helium. Such a refrigerant system could be located at some distance from the scanner and would consume 5–20 kilowatts of power.

Superconductive magnets are permanent magnets in the sense that once the current in them is started the magnet maintains the field without outside power. Other than replenishing their liquid gases and maintaining the vacuum, they should require no major maintenance for several years.

Quench

Superconductivity is a delicate phenomenon and can disappear seemingly without reason. When this happens, the magnet is said to *quench* and the field drops to zero. Fear has been expressed in the past lest a quench occur with a patient in position. Quenches are most likely to happen while technicians are working on the system; a patient is unlikely to be inside during these times. With the advanced design of modern superconductive magnets, a quench is unlikely to be dangerous to a patient in the magnet or a person nearby, because it usually takes more than a few seconds for the field strength to fall to zero. In a recent experiment, an anesthetized pig was subjected to the quench of a 1.7 tesla field. In this experiment, the field collapsed over a period of about 20 seconds, with no evident harm to the animal (Bore, 1986).

In an ordinary quench, the superconductive wire remains intact physically and, as the field collapses, the considerable energy stored in the field is largely dissipated in the coil, heating it and boiling off some or all of the helium. In the unlikely event of a mechanical disaster in which, for example, an earthquake split the gantry open, breaking the coils and spilling much liquid gas, the rapidly collapsing field could, theoretically, cause electrical arcing at unpredictable places, but the major threat to life would probably be asphyxiation from the large volume of inert gases released.

After a total quench, depending on its cause, down time could be several hours to several weeks. The cause must be determined; it is usually some defect in the liquid helium containment. When the cause has been corrected, a substantial fraction, perhaps all 300–500 liters of the helium content of the magnet will likely have to be replaced. After cooling, the build-up of field typically requires several hours.

Quenching of superconductive magnets might be thought of as the MRI equivalent of X-ray tube failure in CT; both are expensive sources of unreliability. Quenching is much rarer than X-ray tube failure, but each quench is more costly.

Field Strength of Superconductive Magnets

These large, stable magnets offer high field strengths and great uniformity of field over an extended period of time. It might be thought that a zero resistance conductor could carry an infinitely large current, but there is a limit on the current any given conductor can carry at a given temperature and field strength. Above this limit, the conductor becomes resistive, causing heating and then quenching. It is entirely practical to make a 2–4 tesla clinical magnet and, indeed, some of the currently installed scanners have a magnet capable of 2 tesla, although they can be run at lower strengths. Whether or not such strong fields will find any wide clinical use is controversial.

Many of the currently available superconductive systems use fields of about 0.35–0.6 tesla, considerably below their rated maximum. This seems to be adequate for high resolution clinical hydrogen imaging.

Federal regulations require that access of the public to all space having field strength of more than five gauss must be controlled. High field magnets require correspondingly larger controlled space. This extensive field outside the gantry, the fringe field, is an inherent disadvantage of either resistive or superconductive electromagnets.

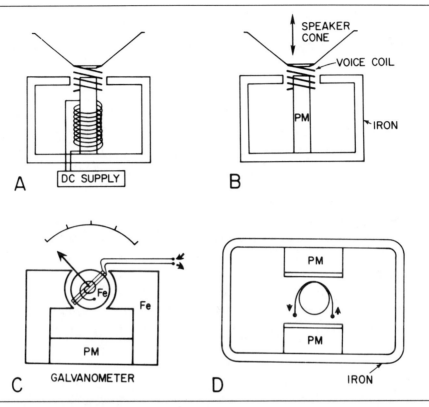

Figure 59. Most modern electronic devices (such as loudspeakers and galvanometers) that require a strong, constant magnetic field use permanent magnets (PM). Before the development of alnico permanent magnets, the strong constant field in a loudspeaker was created by more expensive resistive magnets (A). Figure (D) shows a simplified MRI permanent magnet with excitation coil in place.

PERMANENT MAGNETS

The main magnetic field can be generated by large permanent magnets. The most common magnets in everyday experience, such as compass needles and bar magnets, are examples of permanent magnets. This type of magnetism is based on the property of ferromagnetism, possessed by certain elements, alloys, and ceramic substances. These solids have an electron shell structure such that, when they are placed in a strong external magnetic field, their atoms align with it and remain more or less aligned, even after the external field is removed. The entire solid remains more or less permanently magnetic. The field of this permanent magnet is constant, with no need for a continuous power supply; no heat is generated, and no liquid gases are needed for cooling.

Many everyday electromagnetic devices which require a strong, constant, and inexpensive magnetic field use a permanent magnet to generate this field. Examples of such devices are: loudspeakers, galvanometer movements, and small electric motors (Figure 59).

While permanent magnets are capable of producing magnetic fields of strengths comparable to those of resistive magnet systems, it is difficult to design a permanent magnet which will produce a field with high uniformity over a large enough volume for MRI. Permanent magnet designs have used two magnetic surfaces (pole faces) separated by a gap large enough for a patient. However, simply using two flat pole faces does not produce a magnetic field with high enough uniformity. Since magnetic field lines repel each other much as do electrical charges, they tend to bulge out of any gap in the iron magnetic path unless they are confined by another design feature. Most permanent magnet designs constrict the bulging of the field in order to achieve the desired uniformity, either by shaping the surface of the pole faces or by using weak electromagnets to shim the final field.

Two of the major differences between permanent magnets and electromagnets are in the orientation of the magnetic field through the body and in the amount of fringe field produced by each. In electromagnet (resistive and superconductive) systems, the magnetic field passes longitudinally through the body. Within the imaged volume, the field is uniform: The lines of force are parallel. At the gantry openings, the field spreads out into the room, curving out around the scanner and into the other opening, forming a complete magnetic circuit. The portion of the magnetic field that extends outside the scanner into the surrounding environment is the *fringe field*, which exists because the magnetic field requires a return path to form a complete circuit. In most electromagnets, this return path is entirely through air. An object distorting the field outside the scanner distorts the field inside as well (Figure 60).

In permanent magnets, on the other hand, the magnetic field moves directly between the two pole faces, passing transversely through the patient. The pole faces are mounted on opposite sides of a large rectangular or oval steel frame. The magnetic field goes through the air between the pole faces, through the back of one pole face, through the steel frame, and into the back of the other pole face. Because the return path is almost entirely through the steel frame of the scanner itself, MRI scanners using permanent magnets to generate the main field have very little fringe field (Figure 61).

One permanent magnet unit is commercially available with a field strength of 0.3 tesla (Fonar Corporation). Although this particular design is very heavy (90,000 kilograms), it makes excellent images and requires very little power. It requires no liquid gases and cannot quench. The initial cost is about the same as superconductive scanners, but it has a trivial maintenance cost and, because of its low fringe field, can be installed in a relatively small (but well-supported) space, with few building modifications compared to electromagnets. Importantly, this magnet proves that there are no insurmountable engineering obstacles presented by the proximity (and thus interaction) of the gradient coils and other coil units with the nearby pole faces of the permanent magnet. It is to be hoped that the success of this pioneering magnet will

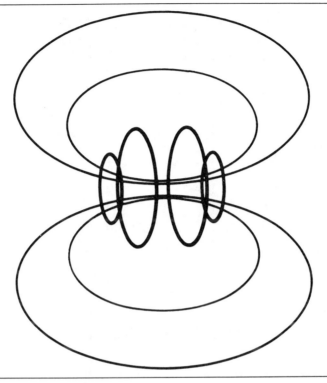

Figure 60. In electromagnets the field spreads out at the gantry openings, forming a return path through the surrounding air and creating fringe field.

encourage further development of permanent magnets — particularly smaller, lighter, and less expensive magnets — to provide the main field. If lighter permanent magnets (3–5 thousand kilograms) were to become available, the major advantages of an MRI system using this design would be: ease of manufacture, low cost, long life without appreciable field loss, low fringe field, minimal maintenance, and no building modifications.

Several manufacturers are currently using permanent magnets in laboratory chemical shift (NMR) spectral analyzers. Each company offers a line of analyzers through a range of quality. At the lower (least expensive) end of each line are usually permanent magnet devices. Unexpectedly high uniformities can be achieved because the sampled volume is so small (less than one cubic centimeter). It is possible that MRI scanners using permanent magnets will become common clinical instruments for many applications other than clinical chemical shift spectroscopy, in which very high field uniformity and strength are essential.

Permanent magnets have the disadvantage, relative to superconductive magnets, that their practical field strength is limited to less than about 1.2 tesla, even if there were no restriction on weight. Permanent magnets have iron in their magnetic circuits, which saturates above this field strength

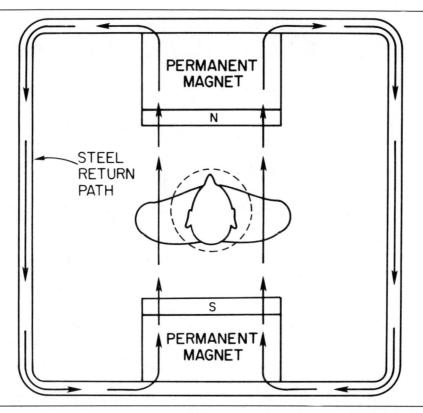

Figure 61. Design of a permanent magnet MRI scanner. Blocks of magnetic material are mounted on opposite sides of a square steel frame. The field passes between the two pole faces and forms a return path through the frame; there is no fringe field. The dashed circle represents the region of high field uniformity, acceptable for imaging.

(Figure 62). Electromagnets can generate much stronger fields because their magnetic return path is air, which does not saturate. In addition to being unable to achieve the strong field offered by air-path superconductive magnets, it is unlikely that any permanent magnet design will produce the high uniformity required for clinical spectroscopy.

WHAT MAGNETIC FIELD STRENGTH IS REQUIRED FOR MRI?
This has been a highly controversial subject, the center of heated discussion since 1983 when marketing of scanners began in earnest. Generally, each manufacturer promotes its own design, and particularly the strength of its main magnet, as best. The debate is usually conducted in terms of *low-field* versus *high-field* MRI scanners, "low-field" being defined as less than about 0.5 tesla, and "high-field" greater than 1 tesla.

In general, because the costs and limitations of main magnet production increase as the field strength increases, the ideal field is the lowest that will do

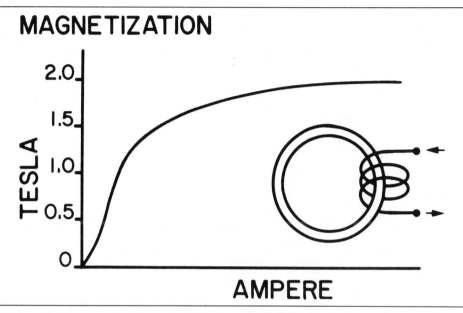

MAGNETIZATION

Figure 62. Current passed through a loop of wire wrapped around a circular piece of iron creates a magnetic field, magnetizing the iron. As current load is increased, the iron becomes more magnetized. But between one and two tesla, the iron becomes saturated and cannot be further magnetized.

the job. Since the "jobs" that MRI will be asked to do have not yet been fully defined, it is impossible to suggest an ideal field strength.

Advantages of High-Field Strength

At higher field strengths, hydrogen nuclei tend to align more and so can absorb more energy. The magnetization vectors for the voxels are larger; the signal from the tissues is correspondingly stronger. This excess signal can be used for more rapid imaging or for other data manipulation.

The fact that the signal strength increases as the field becomes stronger is of particular importance because there is also a constant background noise emitted from the tissues: Thermal motion in the tissues produces a radio signal of its own, consisting of a wide range of frequencies. The amplitude of this noise is independent of the strength of magnetic field applied to the tissues. As the strength of the main field increases, the signal from the hydrogens being imaged increases, while the background thermal noise remains the same: The signal-to-noise ratio increases.

To use an everyday analogy, when we listen to a distant radio station, the radio receiver automatically increases its sensitivity in order to detect the weak signal. But in addition to being more sensitive to the desired signal, the receiver also becomes more sensitive to electrical noise. The station's signal is then difficult to hear because it is mixed with random clicks and hisses, the background noise that comes from many different sources. When we listen to a strong radio station, the receiver's sensitivity automatically decreases, and the background noise is less noticeable. The stronger radio station has a better signal-to-noise ratio.

Stronger fields are also important in hydrogen or phosphorus chemical shift spectroscopy. Each magnetic nucleus in a particular organic molecule is surrounded by a unique cloud of moving electrons. These moving electrons create their own magnetic field which cancels, to a very slight degree, the field strength to which each nucleus is exposed. This slightly lower field causes a lowering of the larmor frequency and this is called *chemical shift*. At lower field strengths it is difficult to separate spectral peaks. At higher field strengths, not only is the signal from any particular peak stronger, but the resonant frequency is increased in proportion to the field strength: Spectral peaks are more spread apart in absolute numbers of cycles per second. This simplifies their electronic separation.

Nuclei of ^{13}C, ^{23}Na, and ^{31}P produce very feeble signals that can be measured only by chemical shift spectroscopy. To produce sharp spectral peaks, a tissue component of possible interest must be freely mobile and unattached to either membranes or large molecules. As a consequence, relatively few substances are identifiable in tissues. In a clinical setting, chemical shift spectroscopy probably will find few applications.

Disadvantages of Strong Magnetic Fields

In general, cost rises with field strength. It is probably impractical to create a resistive magnet stronger than about 0.2 tesla, because of heat dissipation problems. To produce stronger fields, the more expensive superconductive magnets must be used.

The building space dedicated to the scanner rises with field strength, because of the fringe field created by electromagnets. As field strength increases, the acceptable 5 gauss field line moves farther away from the scanner, and site preparation costs rise accordingly. For high-field superconductive magnets, the cost of site preparation can be almost as much as for the scanner itself. The fringe field can be very annoying, in that it will distort television and computer screen images at considerable distances. Many older model video cameras cannot be used within 5–10 meters of the magnet.

Elongated ferromagnetic materials in the body (such as some vascular clips) experience a torque tending to orient them parallel to the field. The torque is proportional to field strength. Fortunately, most metallic prosthetic materials implanted surgically are not significantly ferromagnetic.

Effects on cardiac pacemakers can be expected to be greater at high fields. Pacemaker problems must eventually be solved by redesigning pacemakers, if widespread use of MRI is to be implemented.

High field strengths allow for greater signal strength, but require stronger gradients and, especially, stronger excitation pulses, causing tissue heating.

In high-field machines, typical transmitter power (during a pulse) is about

10 kilowatts, comparable to many radio broadcast transmitters. Although all commercial scanners meet conservative governmental requirements for power deposition, it should be noted that in multiple-echo pulse sequences the transmitter is on a substantial fraction of the time. These pulse sequences require the body to be exposed to a series of strong (180°) radio pulses, each of which may be 1–8 milliseconds long, and repeated 20–50 times per second. In some modern spin-echo imaging, the echo is produced by repeated reversal of the Z-gradient field, rather than by the 180° inverting pulse. The power transmitted into the tissue, and consequent tissue heating, is thereby greatly reduced.

The strong currents intermittently present in the various gradient coils cause them to act like the voice coil in a loudspeaker, so their on-off activity results in a click or thump heard by the patient. With multislice excitation the gradients must be changed many times per second, and this makes a very loud machine-gun like noise which is disturbing to some patients. This gradient coil noise increases with the square of the field strength (assuming a proportionate gradient strength) and undoubtedly contributes to the claustrophobic response of a small percentage of patients.

In strong magnetic fields, the gradients must be proportionately stronger, otherwise chemical shift of signal from fatty tissues causes the image to appear at a different position than the water signal from the same tissue, thereby producing a ghost image. The necessarily precise gradient coil amplifiers must be stronger in high field machines.

The energy stored in the field (which must be dissipated during a quench) rises with the square of field strength. Any ill effects of a quench on patients or the apparatus itself would increase accordingly.

In electromagnets (superconductive and resistive), the spread of the fringe field must be taken into account. In permanent magnets the return path is within the scanner itself; but in resistive and superconductive scanners, it spreads out to include all of the surrounding space. Fortunately, in the first 5–10 meters, the field strength falls off with the inverse cube of distance, rather than inverse square as one might intuitively believe. This means that the field strength falls by a factor of eight rather than four each time the distance from the magnet is doubled.

Where the field converges at the openings of the magnet, large gradients exist. These draw nearby ferromagnetic materials, such as wrenches and gas tanks, into the ends of the gantry. This phenomenon, known as the *missile effect*, is more pronounced at higher field strengths.

In conclusion, one should not judge a scanner solely on the type of magnet used to generate its main field, on the field strength, or on uniformity. Most of the currently available superconductive systems use fields of about 0.35–0.5 tesla, considerably below their theoretical capability. This appears sufficient for high resolution clinical hydrogen imaging. One resistive scanner with a field of only 0.02 tesla is now being marketed. Its ability to produce clinically useful images invites re-evaluation of the entire question of field strength.

If such low-field resistive scanners enjoy continued success, the development of MRI scanners based on small permanent magnets might also be stimulated.

FIELD UNIFORMITY

When discussing field uniformity, both the uniformity of the magnetic field and the volume over which the uniformity is to exist must be stated.

In standard chemical analytic spectrometers, the major practical application since Purcell and Bloch published their discovery of NMR in 1946, the required uniformity is extremely high — less than one part in ten billion — but the volume is extremely small — about five millimeters in diameter. Such extreme uniformity is unnecessary in clinical MRI scanners.

The most stringent requirements for MRI scanning are in chemical shift spectroscopy, which requires about one part in ten million uniformity over a ten centimeter volume. For clinical hydrogen imaging, the requirements are much less strict. Depending upon spatial resolution requirements and the image reconstruction method used, uniformity of one part in ten thousand over a volume of 50 centimeters may be adequate.

As this imaged volume is reduced, any given magnet shows greater field uniformity; more imperfections are likely to be encountered in a larger volume. Although a scanner's field may have a uniformity of one part in a hundred thousand over a 50 centimeter volume (and thus be unacceptable for chemical shift spectroscopy), a small surface (topical) coil might examine only a 5–8 centimeter diameter volume within this region of the total field. Within this smaller volume, the uniformity would be higher, and possibly acceptable for spectroscopy.

There is little reason to be preoccupied with extremely high uniformity for clinical hydrogen imaging as a means of improving image resolution. Clinical MRI seems to be limited to spatial resolution of about 0.5 millimeters, since there is approximately this much movement even in the most cooperative patient, due to heart and respiratory movements.

GRADIENT COILS

Whether the main magnet is superconductive, resistive, or permanent, it generates a constant magnetic field of the required strength and uniformity, throughout the course of the scan, in a volume large enough to be clinically useful. In order for imaging to take place, it is necessary to modify the main field in a controlled and systematic manner, creating magnetic gradients.

These nonuniformities are created by gradient coils housed in the gantry of the scanner. The gradient coils are themselves electromagnets, generating a magnetic field when current is passed through them. Because the gradient fields are so much weaker than the main field, much less power is needed to create them, and heating is not a problem. Because the gradients are switched on and off, current flows only intermittently.

To understand how the MRI scanner uses gradient coils to create magnetic gradients, we might first examine how the current in a single wire interacts with the main field.

Moving electric current in a wire produces a circular magnetic field, expressed graphically as concentric lines (Figure 54). The direction of the magnetic field is determined by the direction of the current, using the right-hand rule. The direction of the field is reversed by changing the direction of the current.

A current-carrying wire placed perpendicular to the main field distorts the field. On one side of the wire, the direction of the wire's own field is the same as the main field: The fields reinforce, and the strength of the total field on that side of the wire is increased. On the other side of the wire, the direction of the gradient coil's field opposes the main field: The fields cancel, and the total field on that side of the wire is decreased (Figures 63A and 63B).

The function of the gradient coils is to use these additions and subtractions to modify the main field, so that its strength changes in a continuous fashion in a desired direction. The coils are circular or semicircular loops of wire. There are three separate sets of gradient coils, each producing a gradient along one of the coordinate axes: X, Y, and Z.

Z-axis Gradient

The longitudinal Z-axis gradient is the most easily understood. It is produced by two circular loops of wire positioned perpendicular to the Z-axis, on either end of the region to be examined (Figure 64). If current is passed in opposite directions in the two loops, clockwise in one and counterclockwise in the other, the field produced by one will add to the main field and the other subtract from it. Between the two loops, the resulting main field will show a gradual transition from a slightly higher field at the adding coil, to a slightly lower field at the subtracting coil. This is the Z-axis gradient.

X and Y Gradients

The Z-axis coils are easily positioned in the gantry, because they conform to the cylindrical patient opening. Pairs of circular coils cannot be used to create gradients in the X and Y axes. Instead, two half circles of wire are used, on opposite sides of the patient.

Two pairs of half circles arranged on the left and right of the patient add and subtract in the X axis, causing an X-gradient. When current is passed in opposite directions in these two half loops, the field from the half loop on the right subtracts from the main field on the right, and the other half loop adds to the main field on the left, creating a gradient in the transverse plane across the patient, with field strength increasing from right to left (Figure 65).

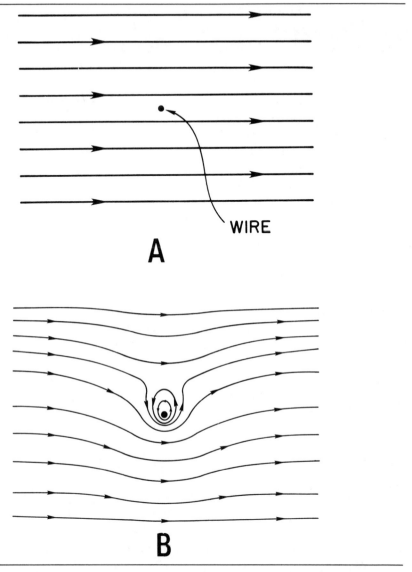

WIRE

A

B

Figure 63A + B. **(A)** Parallel lines of force represent uniformity of the main field. There is no current flowing in the wire, so it does not affect the main field.
(B) A wire carrying current out of the page generates a surrounding magnetic field which interacts with the main field. According to the right-hand rule, the field of the wire opposes (and cancels) the main field above the wire but reinforces the main field below the wire.

Another pair of half loops above and below the patient similarly create the Y gradient.

In an MRI scanner, each of these opposed half loops is paired, and connected with wire running in the Z direction. The straight connecting wires

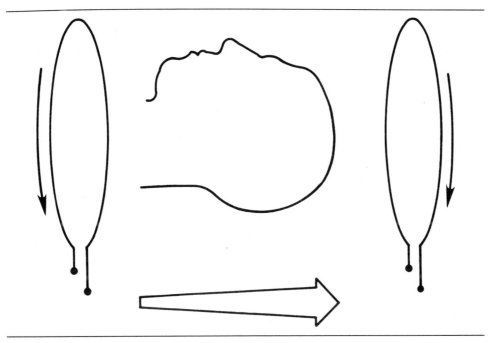

Figure 64. The longitudinal Z-axis gradient is created by two circular coils of wire. Current is passed in opposite directions through the two coils, as shown. The main field is reinforced near the coil on the right and diminished near the coil on the left, resulting in a magnetic gradient between the two coils.

produce no magnetic field component in the Z direction and so do not add to or subtract from the main field. Only the curved portions of coil (in the X-Y plane) are active in creating X and Y gradients. The pairs of curved half circles and the wires connecting them are called *saddle coils* because of their shape (Figure 66).

These saddle coils and the circular Z-axis coils are oriented as shown in Figure 67. When currents are passed through them in the directions shown, the desired gradients are created.

Adding Gradients

Magnetic gradients of any strength can be created independently along any axis by the appropriate pair of coils. Gradients can be expressed mathematically as vectors: The length of the vector indicates the strength of the gradient, that is, the extent of the change in field strength; the orientation of the vector (whether positive or negative along its axis) indicates the direction of the gradient. Two or more gradients in the same region of space combine to form a single gradient.

For example, in the absence of a Z gradient, X- and Y-axis gradients add to form a single gradient in the X-Y plane. By adjusting the relative

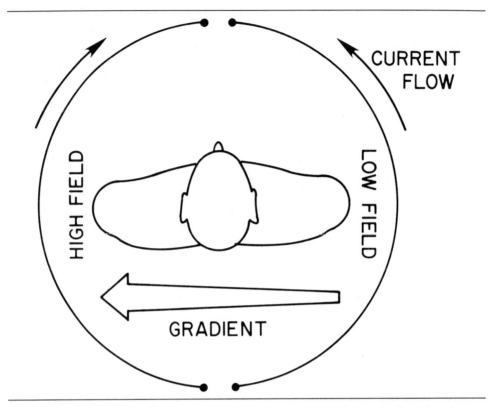

Figure 65. A transverse gradient is created using opposed semicircular loops of wire in which current flows in opposite directions. The field from one semicircular loop adds to the main field, and the field from the other subtracts from it, forming a gradient.

Here, the arrangement for X-axis gradient coils is shown. If the main field has its north pole at the patient's feet and its south at the head, the gradient coils will add to the main field on the left and subtract from it on the right, according to the right-hand rule.

strengths and polarity (up-or-down, left-or-right) of the individual X and Y gradients, a single gradient of any strength and direction in the X-Y plane can be produced, the vector sum of the X and Y gradients.

In Chapter 3, we described the imaging of a transverse slice of tissue: Isolation of this slice of tissue is achieved by applying a Z-axis gradient to the body and exposing it to a pulse of radio-frequency energy of a single wavelength; after the slice has been excited and thus isolated, the Z-axis gradient is turned off. Further localization is obtained by applying a second gradient, this time in the transverse X-Y plane. The direction of the transverse gradient localizes the hydrogen nuclei along a set of parallel lines, perpendicular to the vector representing this gradient.

The direction of this transverse gradient is determined by some combination of strength and polarity of the individual X and Y gradients: The direction of the net X-Y gradient can be rotated progressively like the hands of a clock, by appropriate changes in the strength and polarity of the indi-

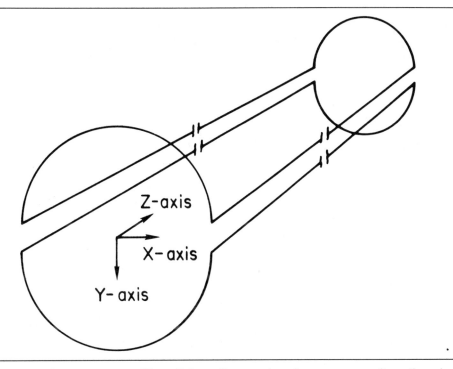

Figure 66. MRI scanners use saddle or Golay coils to produce the transverse gradients (here the arrangement for the Y gradient is shown). Each saddle coil consists of two semicircular loops of wire connected by straight wires. The semicircular portions are active in creating the gradient; the straight portions only serve to connect the loops and do not contribute.

vidual X and Y gradients. Each successive rotation of the gradient localizes the nuclei along a new set of parallel lines.

Other Orientations

While this sequence of gradients (first Z and then X-Y) is used to image a transverse plane, other anatomical planes (sagittal, coronal, etc.) can be imaged with equal facility, by exchanging roles between X, Y, and Z gradients. Since the gradients are controlled electronically, there are no moving parts involved in changing the orientation of the imaged plane, or indeed anywhere in the MRI process. This ease of changing orientation of slice selection is a major advantage over X-ray CT, in which scans are limited to within a few degrees of transverse.

The precision of these gradients must be as good as modern engineering allows. The coils must be physically shaped and positioned with great care and remain stationary during the scanning procedure. The amplifiers supplying their currents must provide exactly the right amount of extremely constant current and must be able to change from one current level to another and become stable at the new level within about one millisecond. Although the controlling voltages, which involve very small currents, are

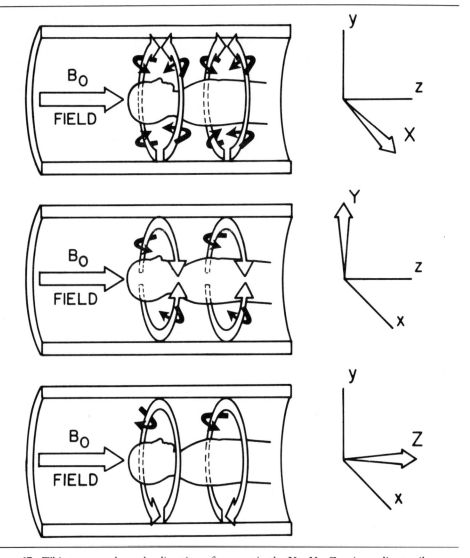

Figure 67. White arrows show the direction of current in the X-, Y-, Z-axis gradient coils; black arrows represent field produced by coils. These fields interact with the main field (B_o), resulting in the gradient along the coordinate axis shown on right.

easy to produce with the required accuracy, the amplifiers required to provide the very large gradient coil currents at low voltage involve a high level of engineering skill.

EXCITATION AND RECEIVING COILS

In order for the hydrogen nuclei to be stimulated during imaging, the tissues must be exposed to energy in the form of a radio signal; the subsequent signal from the tissues must also be detected. These functions are carried out by transmitting and receiving coils contained in a separate unit wrapped closely around the region of the body being imaged.

As discussed in the Appendix, the radio signal, to be most effective, must enter the tissue at right angles to the main field. Since the main field in most scanners is longitudinal, the signal must enter the tissues transversely (in the X-Y plane). A simple wrap-around circular transmitting coil would be ineffective, because it would produce only a longitudinal signal. Instead, a saddle coil is used to produce the transverse signal; in design it is similar but not identical to the saddle coils used to produce the transverse X- and Y-axis gradients.

Saddle-shaped transmitting and receiving coils are used in most commercial scanners because the main field is longitudinal (along the Z-axis). In permanent magnets and at least one experimental resistive unit, the main field is directed transversely (perpendicular) to the body. In such transverse main fields, simple circular coils — rather than saddle coils — are most efficient. Such coils generate a longitudinal radio signal, perpendicular to the transverse main field, providing the most efficient excitation. Similarly, they produce the most efficient reception. Below about 0.3 tesla, such a simple coil will produce about twice the signal of a comparable saddle coil. Above this field strength, the relationship between orientation of antenna and field direction becomes less important.

Because they must be held in precise position, the gradient coils are usually housed in the gantry, separated from the patient compartment. They define the spatial coordinates in the patient. The excitation and antenna coils are placed within the patient compartment and are removable. Commercial concerns offer separate body and head coils, the latter being smaller. It is possible to make one coil serve as both the excitation and receiving antenna, since excitation and detection are not carried out at the same time. With the growing interest in surface coils, which are smaller antenna coils placed directly on various parts of the body, it has become convenient to use separate coils for excitation and receiving: the larger antenna coil can be removed and the surface coil used instead.

SURFACE COILS

Much of the future of magnetic imaging lies in the ability to image small tissue volumes at high resolution. This is accomplished by means of surface antenna coils, which are usually circular copper wire or tubing placed on the surface of the body over the region to be examined.

This circular surface coil defines an approximately spherical volume of space, with the coil itself as the equator of the volume. The coil is a receiving antenna, sensitive to signal emitted from tissues within this volume. Because the hemisphere away from the body contains only air, it produces no signal. All of the signal comes from the other hemisphere, the one containing the tissue to be imaged (Figure 68).

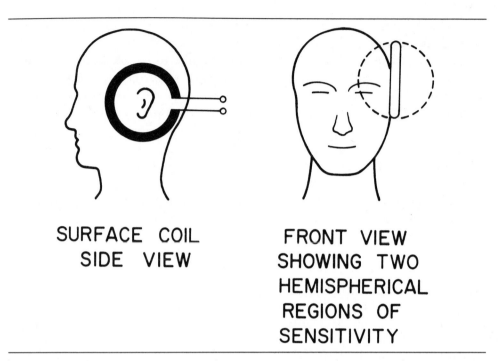

SURFACE COIL
SIDE VIEW

FRONT VIEW
SHOWING TWO
HEMISPHERICAL
REGIONS OF
SENSITIVITY

Figure 68. A surface coil is a small receiving antenna consisting of a circular loop of copper wire or tubing placed on the surface of the body. It detects signal in a spherical volume, but because one hemisphere contains only air, all of the signal comes from the hemisphere of tissue.

Except for the substitution of the surface receiving coil for the full-body receiving coil, the scanning apparatus remains the same. Full-body excitation coils are used, and the procedure for imaging an entire slice is followed. Instead of the signal being received from the entire slice, however, the surface coil detects a signal from only that portion of the excited slice lying within the small hemispherical volume. This is then processed by the computer as though it were the signal from an entire slice.

There are three major advantages of surface coils. First, a small anatomical region is spread over the entire display matrix, thereby improving resolution; this is particularly important in small structures such as the orbit: Spatial resolution is improved by a factor of at least two, compared to scans of the entire slice. Second, the close proximity of the surface coil to the imaged tissue results in a high sensitivity to signal from this small volume. Third, because the surface coil receives signal from only a small volume, there is less thermal noise mixed with the desired image signal: Signal-to-noise ratio and image quality are improved. The surface coil receives signal from only a portion of the slice being imaged and random thermal noise from only the small amount of tissue in the hemispherical volume. In contrast, a saddle-coil receives noise from a very much larger volume of tissue, compared to the slice being imaged.

CHAPTER 7: ADVANTAGES AND LIMITATIONS OF CT

Upon first consideration, MRI seems to be an extension of CT, because MRI sections superficially resemble those made by CT (at least in the transverse plane). An obvious difference, however, is that the inner and outer tables of the skull are black on the MRI scan, while compact bone on the CT scan is white. It would be a mistake to consider MRI as just the next generation CT scanner (Figure: see frontispiece).

The differences between the two types of scans, and the advantages and limitations of each technique, come from the nature of the probes they use, and the hardware needed to produce them. In CT, the probe used is a narrow beam of X-rays. In MRI, the probe consists of magnetic fields used in conjunction with radio energy.

CT scanning has several advantages. The most important of these is CT's short scan time: Scans can be completed in one to five seconds. Unlike MRI, the presence of metallic objects and pacemakers in the patient does not preclude scanning. For these reasons, CT is universally applicable: Essentially all patients can be scanned, except for those that cannot remain motionless for the short duration of the scan. In addition, the theory and application of CT to scanning of patients are both easily comprehended.

CT has been and remains an extremely valuable diagnostic tool. It also has several fundamental limitations: (1) the limited tissue characterization due to the nature of the X-ray probe, (2) restriction of CT scanning to transverse slices due to simple physical constraints and (3) practical limit on numbers of X-rays which can be produced in the short time of the scan.

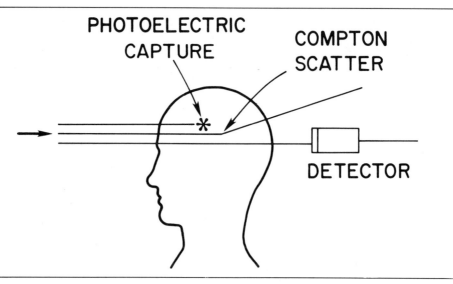

Figure 69. Three X-rays enter the head in the direction of the detector. The bottom X-ray reaches the detector, since it does not interact with the tissues. The upper X-ray collides with and loses all its energy to an atom; this photoelectric capture usually occurs with only very heavy atoms, such as iodine in contrast media. The middle X-ray undergoes a grazing collision with a tissue atom, is deflected a few degrees from its path, and misses the detector; this compton scattering is the most common interaction between diagnostic X-rays and tissue atoms. These two types of interaction are the only sources of tissue characterization in CT.

TISSUE CHARACTERIZATION: SPECIFIC GRAVITY

We commonly think that X-rays are absorbed by tissues. In fact, the atoms which make up the soft tissues of the body are not efficient absorbers of diagnostic X-rays. To actually absorb these X-rays efficiently, an atom must be of a high atomic number. Most of the body's tissue atoms (hydrogen, carbon, oxygen, and nitrogen) are too light to do more than deflect the X-rays away from their original path. This is known as *compton scattering*; in soft tissues it creates a random forward spray of X-rays (Figure 69). On a medical radiograph, the effect of this scattering is to generally fog the film, resulting in poor soft tissue definition.

In CT scanning, however, the scattering of X-rays by soft tissues contributes to the creation of the image. CT uses a narrow beam of X-rays, which follow a precisely defined path between source and detector. When the X-rays are deflected from their original path (by even a small angle), they fail to strike the detector. The deflected X-rays do not fog the image reconstructed by the computer, but leave the imaging process completely. Compton scattering is essentially the only type of interaction between X-rays and tissues (in the absence of contrast media).

The fact that there is only this one interaction means that there is only limited characterization of tissues. Because the number of X-rays undergoing compton scattering is proportional to the mass of the tissue in the path, the CT scan is a map of the specific gravity of tissues.

If one had to choose a tissue characteristic for clinical diagnostic use, one would scarcely choose specific gravity. However, because of the nature of compton scattering, specific gravity is all that is available. This is true not only in CT but in all X-ray images, since they largely represent the scattering of incident X-rays by the tissues being radiographed.

In the case of CT, the ability to image the regional density with considerable precision has produced anatomical correlations which clearly have been of immense clinical usefulness. The modern CT scanner can measure specific gravity to a precision of one tenth of one percent of the density of water. This is one hounsfield unit.

One unique application of CT's ability to measure specific gravity has been the calculation of the brain's net weight during life. The brain is floating in cerebrospinal fluid, buoyed up almost completely; it has not been possible to calculate or measure the net weight of the living brain from its weight after death, because it is then impossible to duplicate the circumstances found during life. From CT measurements, it is possible to estimate that a 1200–1500 gram living brain has a net weight in cerebrospinal fluid of some 15–20 grams.

TISSUE CHARACTERIZATION: IODINE DISTRIBUTION

The preceeding discussion refers to compton scattering of energetic X-rays by the light atoms normally found in brain. If, however, we inject into the patient a considerable quantity of heavier atoms (such as iodine), absorption occurs and the X-ray, in effect, disappears. This adds a second source of information from CT.

The iodine atom contains several electron shells. When an X-ray passes through the atom, it can transfer its entire energy to one of the tightly bound inner K-electrons. The electron is driven out of the atom and comes to rest nearby. This process of photoelectric capture is the reason why, gram for gram, iodine is much more effective at deleting X-rays from the beam than is living tissue. Iodinated contrast media were in common use long before CT appeared and were applied unchanged to this new diagnostic medium.

Although some 40 grams of iodine is injected in contrasted CT scanning, only a very small fraction of this appears in brain and is normally confined to the blood passing through the brain. Iodine allows the contrasted CT scan to show the distribution of blood as well as regions with a defective blood-brain barrier, where the iodine has leaked out of the blood into the brain extracellular tissue space. About 20% of brain volume is extracellular fluid, so there is a substantial anatomical compartment into which iodine can disperse.

The contrasted scan is a composite of the uncontrasted specific gravity map (from the scattering of X-rays by the body's soft tissue atoms), onto which is superimposed the distribution of the injected iodine. On the contrasted CT image, blood in large vessels becomes much brighter; non-neural tissues become generally brighter, as the iodine distributes in their blood content and in interstitial extracellular fluid. Since the iodinated benzoates are excreted by renal glomerular filtration, the iodine content of the renal medulla and urinary outflow tract rises quickly. In healthy brain tissues, iodine remains confined to blood, because of the blood-brain barrier.

In the uncontrasted scan, the image of density can be obtained without discomfort or hazard, but with the introduction of iodine the procedure is converted from harmless to mildly invasive.

BLOOD-BRAIN BARRIER

In non-neural tissues, there is a free exchange of substances between capillary and interstitial extracellular fluid, because there are gaps between the endothelial cells making up the capillary wall. But in brain and spinal cord, the walls of the capillaries are structurally unique and only selectively permeable. To most charged molecules, they are very impermeable.

Modern water-soluble contrast media are salts and are thus ionized in solution. As a result, in healthy brain, contrast material is confined to blood; this allows some of the larger vessels to be imaged easily. The entire brain, but especially gray matter (with its greater blood volume) lightens perceptibly as the iodine distributes throughout the body in the first 30–60 seconds after injection. In regions of brain which are abnormal for any reason (tumor, trauma, etc.), the brain cannot maintain the selective permeability of its capillaries. In these lesions, iodine leaks through the now-permeable capillaries and achieves a high regional tissue concentration. Consequently, the lesion brightens visibly against the relatively dark background of the surrounding healthy brain.

The contrasted scan can also be compared to a radionuclide scan. The pertechnetate ion ($^{99m}TcO_4^-$), used since 1964 in radionuclide brain scanning, distributes in much the same way as iodinated contrast media. The radionuclide scan, formed from the detection of gamma rays emitted by Tc^{99m}, produces an image of pertechnetate ion distribution. Supplementing the CT scan by injecting contrast medium superimposes on the uncontrasted CT scan an image which is very similar to the radionuclide scan, but of much higher spatial resolution.

NEED FOR CONTRAST INJECTION

In the very early days of CT scanning, the resolution was so poor (an 80×80 display matrix was used) and statistically noisy, that extra lesion enhancement was obtained by injecting the patient with a large intravenous dose of iodinated contrast material. The defective blood-brain barrier and increased blood content in various lesions (notably tumors) caused them to become much more visible.

As CT image quality improved (it has been essentially constant since 1982), so much more detail became visible on the uncontrasted scan that it became rare to find a lesion on the contrasted scan when the uncontrasted scan had been entirely normal. Unfortunately, the practice of routinely contrasting patients had become firmly established, although the need for it had largely passed; it remains commonplace to inject all patients being scanned unless there is a known previous reaction to iodides or there is patient objection. A decision to use contrast should be made only after viewing the uncontrasted scan; if this were done, many fewer patients would be contrasted.

The generally accepted death rate from modern intravenous contrast agents is of the order of one death in 15,000 to 20,000 injected patients. Although this seems an "acceptably" low risk, contrast injection converts the CT scan from an innocuous procedure to one in which all injected patients are made uncomfortable, about one in 1000 will become seriously transiently ill, and about one in 15,000 to 20,000 will die.

From a calculation of the number of CT scans done in the past decade and the portion of those receiving contrast injection, it can be estimated that there have been more than 1000 deaths in the U.S. alone from CT contrast injection. But they occur so rarely that no one institution is likely to collect any significant number of deaths. As a result, deaths from CT are very much under-reported in the routine medical literature. This estimate points out the need for a conservative approach to contrast agents, restricting their use to those patients who are seriously suspected of actual brain pathology, as determined from their clinical history, examination, and review of the un-contrasted scan. In a conservative laboratory, about 25% of patients scanned should receive contrast.

SUMMARY OF CT TISSUE CHARACTERIZATION

These two interactions — scattering and capture of X-rays — are the only sources of information in CT. They give specific gravity of the tissues and distribution of iodine, respectively. While clinically valuable, these are the only available sources of tissue characterization; of these two data sources, the iodine distribution requires physical invasion of the patient.

TRANSVERSE ORIENTATION OF SCAN

The X-ray source and detector are located in the gantry of the CT scanner, on opposite sides of the body. Because of these hardware limitations, CT scanning is restricted to imaging of transverse slices of the body; although by proper positioning of the patient and tilting of the gantry, sections within perhaps 30° of transverse can also be imaged.

It is possible to create coronal or sagittal CT scans by reconstructing them from transverse images. Many very thin transverse sections must first be made; the computer assembles rows of voxels from adjacent slices to create what appears to be a tissue section in a plane other than the one originally scanned. One of the disadvantages of this approach is that imaging of these many thin sections increases patient irradiation, and time of examination is greatly extended. These indirectly reconstructed odd planes are always lower in resolution than the directly scanned transverse sections from which they were made.

In an MRI scanner, the orientation of the cross section is determined by the strengths and directions of the gradient fields within the scanner. Manipulation of these gradients is accomplished electronically, without moving parts, with the consequence that MRI can image in any plane desired. The ability of MRI to create images of equally good resolution in any plane is an enormous advantage of this newer technique.

ANATOMICAL REGIONS INACCESSIBLE TO CT

In imaging, it is the soft tissues that are generally of interest, so CT is most useful in regions in which the volume of soft tissue is large relative to bone and the thickness of surrounding bone is uniform. In these regions, the CT X-ray beam will pass through only a minimal amount of bone, so the effect of soft tissues on the beam is maximized and their image correspondingly improved.

Because the cranial part of the skull is relatively uniform, CT is effective in imaging much of the brain. However, CT is less useful in anatomical regions where soft tissues of interest are surrounded by much bone, particularly when the bone is irregular and consequently projects many fine but intense shadows.

In such regions, the X-ray beam must traverse a large amount of bone. The compton scattering by bone overwhelms that by soft tissues. If the bony region is irregular, the path length in the bone may vary considerably; in such irregular regions, adjacent beam paths pass through widely varying amounts of bone. These factors interfere with the acquisition of information about soft tissue.

Thus the posterior fossa shows poor brain contrast. The fourth ventricle is the most prominent structure seen consistently. Similarly, the entire spinal cord is not well seen. This small structure, suspended in cerebrospinal fluid, is surrounded by very irregular, bony vertebral bodies. When such a structure is scanned, there are very large differences in the amount of bone that adjacent beam paths must pass through before and after they have traversed the spinal canal and the cord inside.

The pituitary in the sella turcica is of great interest, but its usually small size and its complex bony environment make it quite inaccessible by CT. Attempts at tilting the head back sharply to make a near-coronal CT section have been largely unsatisfactory. Many patients cannot achieve or maintain the very awkward position, and the many tangential X-ray paths through the maxillary bone, teeth, and dental fillings cause prohibitive streak artifacts in the brain, and particulary in the pituitary. Similar artifacts are seen radiating from any metal that lies in the tissue section.

The interpetrous space, occupied largely by the pons, is especially inaccessible. Not only is there a great deal of dense bone laterally in the petrous portion of the temporal bone, which absorbs a large fraction of the X-rays the computer needs to compute the intracranial soft tissues, but the many irregular mastoid air cells surrounded by bone cast strong shadows through the interpetrous space.

TISSUE METAL ARTIFACTS

Metallic artifacts within the body create streak artifacts on the final scan by absorbing X-rays much more than surrounding tissues. These metallic objects may seriously interfere with CT scanning, but only if they lie within the plane under examination. Adjacent sections not containing the metallic artifact appear entirely normal. This is unlike MRI, in which a ferromagnetic object of small dimensions may obliterate an entire anatomical region in all directions from the metal. Since shrapnel and other small pieces of steel will likely be present in a small percentage of all patients, and it is not clear how MRI can avoid this artifact. CT has a very great advantage in such cases.

EVOLUTION OF CT SCANNERS

First generation CT scanners such as were originally built by EMI Ltd. under the direction of their inventor, G.N. Hounsfield, used a single narrow beam of X-rays. The X-ray source and detector were positioned on opposite sides of the body and were moved simultaneously in a translation motion so that measurements were taken along a set of parallel lines. Then the entire X-ray source-detector assembly was rotated, and another pass was made across the section from a slightly different angle. This was translate, rotate CT scanning.

The single rectangular beam (about 2.5 centimeters long and about 2 millimeters wide at the middle of the head) was passed through the head to two detectors, each of which saw approximately one half of the 2.5 centimeter length of the cross section of the beam. This allowed two adjacent 1.25 centimeter thick slices of tissue to be examined simultaneously by processing the signal from the two detectors separately. Imaging two adjacent slices simultaneously reduced the total scan time, which was over four minutes for each pair of slices.

Second generation scanners used approximately 30 independent beams which fanned out from their source through a sheet of lead containing 30 collimating holes. Each of these beams was directed at its own detector. The X-ray source and detectors were still moved in a translate-rotate pattern, as

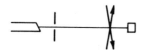

SINGLE BEAM
ROTATE – TRANSLATE

<u>I st GENER</u>

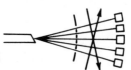

MULTIPLE BEAM
ROTATE – TRANSLATE

<u>2nd GENER</u>

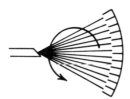

ALL ROTATE
NO TRANSLATION
<u>3rd GENER</u>

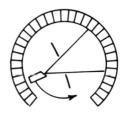

MULTIPLE STATIONARY
CRYSTALS
MOVING X–RAY TUBE

<u>4th GENER</u>

Figure 70. As the design of CT scanners evolved, the relation of the X-ray source to the detector was changed. In first and second generation scanners, both the source and detector moved in translational, as well as rotational motion. In third generation, the translational motion was eliminated; both source and detectors revolved about the patient. In fourth generation, detectors were fixed and only the source moved.

in the first generation, but by using many more beam paths simultaneously a much larger fraction of the generated X-rays was used. This allowed scan times to be reduced from about four minutes (for two slices) in first generation to about 20 seconds (for one slice) in second generation.

In the first two generations of CT scanners, both translation and rotation were separate motions achieved through physical displacement of X-ray source and detectors. Translational motion, in particular, was cumbersome to produce, and this kept the scan time from further shortening. Since the only requirement of CT scanning is to pass the collimated beam through the section many times from many directions, translational motion was unnecessary and was eliminated in later scanners, which used a broad beam and many hundreds of detectors. The beam paths required were created simply by rotation. In third generation scanners, both source and detectors revolve about the patient, in fourth generation only the source moves (Figure 70).

It might easily be inferred that fourth generation CT scanners are superior to third, but both types of scanners are marketed simultaneously and differences in images are not discernable.

PRACTICAL LIMITATIONS OF CT

By 1985, development of new CT scanners had virtually ceased; there was no obvious direction in which to proceed. Scan times were down to a few seconds, and image processing was so fast relative to patient handling times that no further advance seemed worthwhile. Resolution was better than 0.5 millimeters for bone/water contrast; this is probably the practical limit of any scanning method, due to inevitable patient movement from heart action, respiration, and involuntary movements.

Ironically, the X-ray tube itself, which in principle has not changed since the time of Roentgen, remains the weak link in modern CT scanners. To produce a short scan time, many X-rays must be produced per unit time. This requires very high beam currents, which push anode heat dissipation to extremes. It is common to replace two to three X-ray tubes per year. These are only partially covered by machine warranty and not at all by service contract. After the warranty period, each X-ray tube replacement can be expected to cost $15,000–20,000 and to result in about one day of downtime. When it will occur is not always predictable.

FUTURE OF CT

Despite these limitations, CT has revolutionized the clinical diagnosis and management of head trauma, subdural hematoma, brain atrophy, strokes (particularly with hemorrhagic components), and many other focal and general neurological diseases. Because both CT and MRI have several unique limitations at present, they will usefully complement each other for a time. There should, because of the safety and extended tissue characterization possible with MRI, be a gradual shift toward magnetic studies and, very likely, a nearly complete replacement of X-rays for diagnostic purposes by the end of the century.

CHAPTER 8: ADVANTAGES AND DISADVANTAGES OF MRI

Due to the nature of the magnetic probe used in MRI, this technique possesses several fundamental advantages: (1) tissue can be characterized in a number of ways, (2) any plane can be imaged, (3) bone is invisible, so all anatomic regions can be examined, (4) no contrast medium is required, and (5) there is no ionizing radiation.

At the present time, there are also several disadvantages: (1) the complexity and high cost, (2) the long scan time, (3) the noise and isolation experienced by patient during scan, and (4) the exclusion of a substantial fraction of patients due to pacemakers, metallic artifacts, and inability to cooperate. The first three of these are under active development, and improvement can be expected. However, gradient coil noise, pacemakers, and metallic artifacts are more fundamental problems for which solutions are not yet apparent.

INVISIBILITY OF BONE IN MRI

X-rays interact strongly with bone. As a result, bone appears bright on CT scans, and imaging of certain anatomical regions, such as the base of the brain and the spinal cord, is limited. However, bone does not interact with the magnetic fields and radio signals used in MRI. Compact bone is essentially invisible, and even fatty bone marrow can be imaged and indeed is the only bone structure visible.

Earlier in this book, we learned that MRI involves several steps: (1) creation of carefully controlled magnetic fields in the region to be imaged,

(2) exposure of tissue to pulses of radio waves, (3) detection of the signal subsequently emitted from the tissues, and (4) processing of this signal by a computer to reconstruct the final image.

Bone has low magnetic susceptibility, so it does not distort the magnetic fields created by the scanner; soft tissues experience the same magnetic field regardless of the density or shape of adjacent bone. Bone does not interact with the strong radio signal transmitted into the body. The signal from the soft tissues, which is detected by the MRI scanner's antenna, is thus unaffected by nearby or surrounding bone.

The signal from which the scan is made comes largely from hydrogen nuclei of water molecules in soft tissues. Soft tissues have a very high water content, and because much of the water is in liquid form, it is mobile and can be imaged. The signal from compact bone is much weaker for several reasons. First, the water content of compact bone is only about 14%, a fraction of that in most soft tissues. While water in soft tissues is relatively mobile, most of the water in bone is probably bound into the bony crystalline structure as water of hydration and so behaves as a solid, having a very short T_2 (about one millisecond). With this short T_2, the nuclei are completely dephased within ordinary times-to-echo of 20–40 milliseconds. This, together with the low water content, appears to be the major reason for lack of any readable signal from bone. All of the radio signal in MRI is, then, from soft tissues.

While the loss of the usual radiographic bony landmarks is at first disorienting, it soon becomes evident that this is a great advantage. Even structures embedded in bone (such as the pituitary, spinal canal, or posterior fossa contents) can be clearly visualized. The absence of bone in the MRI scan offers the first opportunity to study all of the bone marrow. Since essentially all bones contain marrow, a postmortem anatomical study of all marrow would be tedious in the extreme and probably has never been done. One of the fundamental contributions of MRI could be comprehensive studies of marrow in all of the bones to seek out possible regional abnormalities.

ABILITY TO SCAN ANY PLANE

MRI can directly scan any plane desired. While CT requires physical movement of the X-ray source about the patient, thus restricting imaging to horizontal sections, in MRI the gradient magnetic fields that define the orientation of the plane being imaged are changed electronically, and any plane through the body can be studied. The fact that the quality of these MRI scans in various planes is the same is an enormous advantage in clinical interpretation.

TISSUE CHARACTERIZATION: T_1, T_2, AND MOVEMENT

The most important advantage of MRI is its ability to provide tissue characterization beyond simple hydrogen distribution. By changing the pulse-sequencing used and the computer software, tissue characteristics can be explored from several vantage points. The major tissue characteristics currently being exploited are: T_1, T_2, fluid movement (particularly of blood), and magnetic tissue susceptibility, in addition to water hydrogen distribution.

In Chapter 4, we introduced the principles of tissue characterization. There are two aspects of the behavior of the hydrogen nucleus that can easily be measured by MRI. These are the *time constants* or *relaxation times* T_1 and T_2. By analogy to compasses, we stated that the time constant T_1 indicates the rate at which dephasing of the oscillatory motion of the nuclei takes place. rate at which dephasing of the oscillatory motion of the nuclei take place. These nuclear properties are not in themselves of interest, but they are strongly influenced by the molecular environment of the hydrogen nuclei and can be used as means of characterizing tissues.

The T_1 and T_2 of pure water, at ordinary field strengths, are both about 2.7 seconds. In tissues, both are shorter, with T_2 being much shorter than T_1. Tissue T_1 is about 150–2000 milliseconds, while tissue T_2 is about 20–120 milliseconds. The reasons for the shorter relaxation times of tissue relative to pure water, and of differences in tissue relaxation times between different tissues, are not clear, but some generalizations can be made. The water in tissue cells has a much greater microviscosity than pure water, because it is exposed to many macromolecules and membranous surfaces. These serve to slow down thermal motion of water molecules and thus to accelerate T_1 relaxation. In addition, there are many trace paramagnetic substances, such as dissolved gaseous oxygen, which shorten both T_1 and T_2. Elaborations of these relationships between cellular function, structure, and relaxation times is now under intensive study, and this subject will undoubtedly become considerably clarified.

Most modern scans present a mixture of T_1 and T_2; the degree to which a scan is weighted towards T_1 or T_2 is dependent on the exact pulse sequence used, that is, on the strengths of the individual pulses and the timing between them.

The direction, steepness, and duration of the gradient fields used during the scan is another variable.

T_1-emphasized scans, which often use the inversion-recovery sequence, show excellent gray/white matter differentation and high spatial resolution. When T_1 of a region is long, T_2 of that region is usually long also. Usually, T_2-weighted images better demonstrate brain pathological lesions.

The relationship of relaxation times to image brightness can be confusing. On T_1-weighted scans, regions of short T_1 usually appear bright, while those of long T_1 appear dark. Body fat, for example, has a short T_1 and appears bright on T_1-weighted scans. Its rapid T_1 relaxation prepares it to absorb a great deal of energy from the next excitation pulse. Consequently, its signal is stronger and its image is bright immediately after this next excitation. The shortening of tissue T_1 by paramagnetic contrast agents causes a brighter image for the same reason. Regions of long T_1, such as cerebrospinal fluid, retain their energy longer, do not absorb as much energy from the next excitation pulse, and so appear darker.

On T_2-weighted scans, regions of short T_2 appear dark, and those of long T_2 bright. One advantage of a T_2-weighted scan is that it presents lesions of long T_2 as bright spots on a dark background. In any black and white picture, a bright object of interest on a dark background is more striking than a dark object on a lighter background. Many lesions (for example, cerebral metastases, brain edema, and multiple sclerosis lesions) have a longer T_2 than adjacent healthy brain. In the T_2-weighted scan, the multiple cerebral white matter lesions of multiple sclerosis appear as bright spots in the surrounding darker white matter. T_1-weighted images, on the other hand, usually show these lesions as less obvious dark spots on a field of grayish-appearing white matter. Whichever weighting is used, MRI shows multiple sclerosis lesions with a much greater sensitivity than does CT.

It requires much experience to interpret scans made with various pulse sequences, because so many apparently different images can be made of the same scan slice, depending on the pulse sequence used. The resulting images may look as though they were tissue slices stained with entirely different histological methods. It is best to become familiar with a few pulse sequences and not try to tailor each scan to each patient.

Earlier presentation of pulse sequencing (Chapter 5) should be referred to in order to explore this in more depth.

The accuracy of in vitro relaxation measurements, even in the laboratory, is much worse than one might expect; it is influenced by several obvious variables, such as temperature and oxygen content. Other sources of variability are difficult to pinpoint; estimates of relaxation times from MRI scanners seem to show a wide range for the same tissue in different patients, and even in the same patient upon repeated scans. While gross changes in relaxation times aid in visual interpretation of scans, it would be very useful if accurate and reproducible numbers could also be attached to various regions of the scan. At present, attempts to do so have been disappointing. The literature of this confusing subject has been summarized by P. A. Bottomley (1985).

Imaging of Moving Blood

The entire MRI process presupposes that the nuclei being imaged will be in the same location throughout the sequence of excitation and subsequent re-emission of energy, but blood is moving at a surprisingly rapid rate. In the ascending aorta, as it leaves the heart, its velocity approaches one meter per second. The arteries branch repeatedly; on average they increase their total cross-sectional area by about 25% at each branching, and the velocity of blood slows accordingly. By the time it has reached a capillary, it is moving about 1 millimeter per second; in major arteries in the brain, its velocity is perhaps 10 centimeters per second. This means that in even the brief interval between pulses, the blood has travelled a substantial distance. It no longer

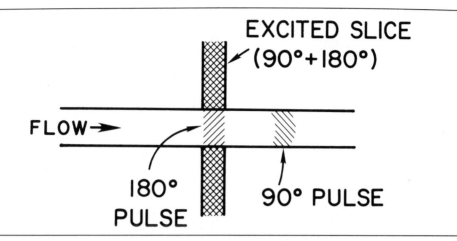

Figure 71. Blood moving rapidly, perpendicular to the plane of excitation, is not in the plane for both pulses of a pulse sequence. Since the same hydrogen nuclei must experience both pulses to produce an echo, and be imaged, moving blood produces very little signal (and so appears black).

responds to pulse sequences as does the adjacent, stationary tissue (Figure 71).

There are several reasons why blood appears black: (1) If moving nearly perpendicular to the plane of section, the same blood may not receive both the 90° and 180° pulses required for the spin echo. (2) If moving substantially parallel to the plane of section, it will have moved into a new region of both the main and gradient fields, having different field strengths; the spin echo process will be largely curtailed, since the 180° pulse inversion requires a constant field nonuniformity to allow refocusing of the echo. (3) Blood flowing in a vessel moves faster in the center than it does near the walls. This results in a continuous slippage of layers of blood between the center of the stream and the wall. The velocity profile is approximately parabolic (Figure 72). Although this blood is subject to the same thermal motion as stationary tissues, there is a superimposed rotation of water molecules caused by their laminar flow, which further accelerates dephasing. (4) Turbulent flow (such as in narrowed vessels), with its multiple vortices and changes in direction, is still another source of dephasing (Figure 73). The latter three sources of dephasing are random and contribute to what is essentially a very short T_2.

In the cerebrospinal fluid cisterns at the base of the brain and in the aqueduct of Sylvius, there are substantial tidal movements due to changes in brain volume, from cardiac action and changes in central venous pressure. These movements of the cerebrospinal fluid are sufficiently fast that they can be imaged and they may become a useful diagnostic aid in space-occupying lesions in the posterior fossa, since these masses could interfere with normal tidal movements. These movements cause some regions of the cerebrospinal fluid to be darker than others.

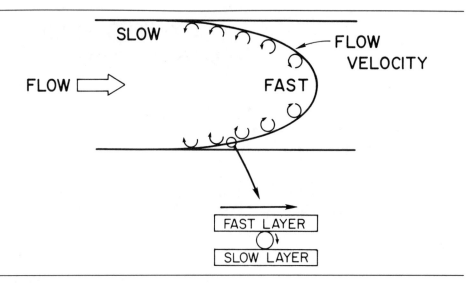

Figure 72. Blood moves faster near the center of the vessel than near the wall. Small arrows show slippage of layers of blood between the center of the vessel and wall. This laminar blood flow further contributes to the lack of signal from moving blood.

It is reasonable to expect that most, or perhaps all, invasive arteriography will eventually be supplanted by noninvasive MRI visualization of vessels.

To summarize, there are currently four clinically useful tissue characteristics which MRI can define: (1) regional hydrogen concentration, (2) regional T_1 behavior, (3) regional T_2 behavior, and (4) regional rate of bulk hydrogen movement (from one location to another). Undoubtedly, many other influences on hydrogen magnetic relaxation in tissues will be measured in the future.

CONTRAST MEDIA

There is so much tissue characterization already available from a modern MRI scan that it is only occasionally that one would wish to introduce contrast material in order to obtain further information, particularly if it could on rare occasion be toxic. The most widely researched contrast media are paramagnetic substances. Paramagnetic substances are atoms that are magnetic due to the structure of their outer electron shells, rather than of their nucleus. In even trace (micromolar) tissue concentrations, paramagnetic substances greatly shorten T_1 and T_2.

Ordinary diatomic O_2 is promising since it can be administered by inhalation for short periods of time, with no concern for its toxicity. O_2 dissolved in tissue water is strongly paramagnetic, while covalently bonded oxygen (as in the water molecule) is not. Inhalation of 100% O_2 brings about a slightly shorter T_1 and T_2 in most regions of the body. This could be useful in detecting areas of reduced blood flow if clinical measurements of T_1 and T_2 become accurate enough to allow these slight changes to be seen.

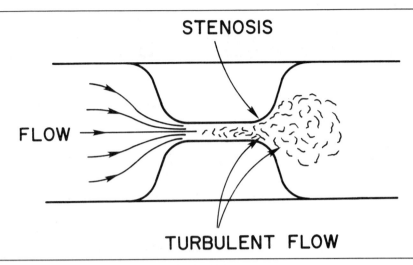

STENOSIS

FLOW →

TURBULENT FLOW

Figure 73. Turbulent blood flow causes increased tumbling and signal loss beyond that due to smooth laminar flow.

Some of the transitional metals such as iron, copper, manganese, and gadolinium are strongly paramagnetic, usually in their reduced (Fe^{+++}, Cu^{+++}, Mn^{+++}) state, and can be chelated with EDTA or DTPA to allow rapid renal clearance. In brain MRI, these chelates behave much like iodinated agents in CT in that, being polar molecules, they achieve substantial concentrations in brain only in blood vessels and in tissues in which the blood–brain barrier is defective.

Although the paramagnetic agents studied to date seem to be nontoxic, rare idiosyncratic reactions can be expected. Whenever there is an intravenous injection, there is the remote possibility that, due to human error, some unintended harmful substance might be injected.

It should be recalled that CT contrast agents were called into use in very early development of CT to make lesions more prominent in the face of very poor resolution. There is so much tissue characterization and high resolution anatomical detail already available with MRI without injecting anything, that there is not the pressure to develop artificial enhancement agents as there was with CT. Whether the development of any of these agents is commercially viable in the presence of a limited market and governmental safety hurdles remains to be seen.

Because contrast media are not required to provide tissue characterization, and because MRI does not even produce the very slight tissue ionization of CT, it is, by comparison, "super safe."

TISSUE HEATING

Because MRI does not use X-rays, there is no possibility of tissue ionization. However, some tissue heating occurs, due partly to rapidly changing gradient fields, but mostly to radio-frequency excitation energy. A very small fraction of the radio-frequency energy pumped into the tissues is absorbed by resonant nuclei; most absorbed energy simply sets up currents in the tissue, thus generating heat.

Particularly for body scans of heavy patients, much power is required to produce 90° pulses and, especially, 180° pulses. It is largely concern over tissue heating that limits the elaboration of pulse sequences and the tissue characterization obtained from them: The number of radio-frequency pulses transmitted into the tissues per unit time is limited. The main field strength of a scanner is a factor: With high field strength machines, stronger excitation pulses are needed, and tissue heating is correspondingly greater.

SERIAL SCANS

The safety of MRI versus CT scanning is demonstrated in development laboratories where technical personnel commonly use their own body as a phantom to test a scanner, perhaps hundreds of times. In clinical practice, one would not hesitate to do as many MRI scans as indicated. No prudent person would use their own body repeatedly as a CT phantom, because of the cumulative effects of ionizing radiation; an inanimate phantom is invariably used in CT. (To our knowledge, the maximum number of CT scans in any one patient is 29.)

In summary, MRI seems to be the most versatile imaging probe yet introduced into medicine. It has an unprecedented ability to characterize tissues, and it appears entirely harmless.

LIMITATIONS OF MRI

At the present time, a substantial fraction of patients cannot be scanned by MRI. Long scan time, confinement, and noise cause enough patient discomfort that only cooperative and alert patients can be scanned successively. These problems are being researched and will undoubtedly be designed out of future MRI scanners. Problems with pacemakers and metallic artifacts are, however, more intractable.

Gantry Size and Confinement

Superficially, the MRI gantry looks like a CT gantry, because both have cylindrical patient spaces. But upon closer inspection, we can see that the MRI gantry is quite different. The most obvious difference is in the depth of the patient space: In most MRI systems, which use resistive or superconductive magnets, the patient space is much longer than that of the CT scanner. In an MRI scanner, the patient space is on the order of two meters; its diameter is one half to one third its length (Figure 74).

The dimensions of the gantry are dictated by the size and placement of the several coils needed to produce the magnetic fields used in MRI. This size and shape is important in patient management in that the anatomical

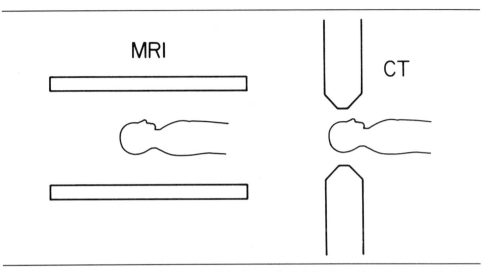

Figure 74. In a CT scanner (right), the patient experiences little discomfort, due to the shallow gantry, low noise, and short scan time. In an MRI scanner (left) the patient is placed in a long cylinder. His sense of confinement is exacerbated by the loud machine gun-like noise and long scan time.

region to be examined must occupy the center of this cylindrical volume. Particularly if the region being imaged is the head, the patient may experience a considerable sense of isolation. After a long period of confinement, totalling perhaps an hour, a substantial fraction of patients become significantly anxious and claustrophobic. Occasionally, patients will look at the deep space in which they are to be confined and refuse to be placed in scanning position.

The isolation also makes it difficult to monitor the ill patient who could experience vomiting, respiratory distress, or unnoticed movement, in addition to the emotional reactions discussed above.

No ferromagnetic support apparatus, such as tanks of gas, can be allowed inside the gantry opening since they will distort the field, ruining the necessary field homogeneity. They might even be pulled from the patient by the scanner's magnetic field. Fortunately, most modern venous infusion apparatus, pharyngeal airways, etc., are made of plastic and aluminum and so do not interact with the field.

Long Scan Time

In 1987, the usual scan period during which the subject must remain immobile was between about 5 and 15 minutes. This is, at present, the most limiting of the disadvantages of magnetic imaging. The throughput of patients (the number that can be examined per day) is considerably less than with CT.

Why is the scan time so long?

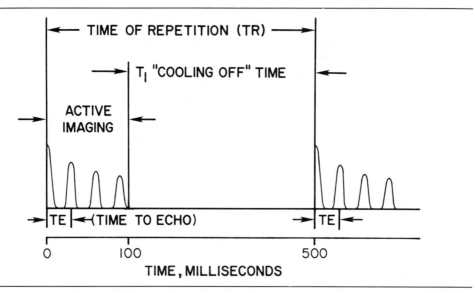

Figure 75. Most of the information from which an MRI scan is reconstructed is contained in the series of echoes which occur within the 100 milliseconds of a pulse sequence. Most imaging uses repeated pulse sequences; before the sequence can be repeated, a considerable amount of time is required to allow T_1 energy loss (cooling off time). This greatly lengthens scan time.

In MRI, the tissues are exposed to brief pulses of radio-frequency energy, each a few milliseconds in length, resulting in stimulation of hydrogen nuclei. A substantial period of time (0.5–2.0 seconds) must be allowed to elapse in order for the nuclei to dissipate their energy and for the tissue to again be receptive to the energy in another pulse.

In most MRI imaging, the tissues are stimulated by a sequence of pulses, rather than just a single pulse. The tissues are exposed to a staccato burst of several radio-frequency pulses. The series of stimulating pulses, and the subsequent re-emitted signals and echoes from which T_2-weighted MRI scans are reconstructed, occur in a period of about 100 milliseconds. After a pause of perhaps 0.5–2.0 seconds, the series of pulses is repeated. This waiting period must be provided to allow the nuclei to relax to the resting, low-energy state they possessed before stimulation (Figure 75).

Most of the time spent in imaging of a single slice of tissue is dead time, during which the nuclei are cooling off. For this reason, MRI scanning is quite lengthy.

One approach that has been taken to shortening scan time has been multi-slice imaging. Instead of completing the imaging of one slice of tissue before moving on to image the next slice, modern scanners image several (perhaps 15) adjacent slices in the same scan sequence. By using appropriate excitation frequencies, adjacent slices are stimulated in rapid sequence; while previously excited slices are relaxing, the scanner is stimulating the next slice. By the time the scanner has finished stimulating the last slice, the first has returned to its prestimulation state and can again be stimulated. Multi-slice techniques were a major advance in shortening scan time.

Another approach which produces an image of lesser quality in a very short time (a few seconds) is the flash scan technique. Here, low-energy pulses producing a vector tipping of only perhaps 10–20 degrees are applied in rapid sequence with perhaps a time of repetition (TR) of 10–50 milliseconds.

Gradient Coil Noise

A conducting metal, immersed in a magnetic field, is subjected to a force when current is passing through it. This is the basis of electric motors and audio loudspeakers. In the latter, intermittent electric current results in the movement of the voice coil and speaker cone, and the consequent production of sound.

The gradient coils, housed within the gantry of the MRI scanner, lie within the larger main field coils and so are subjected to the intense main field. To generate the gradient magnetic fields needed for imaging, electric current must be passed through the gradient coils. This current of electrons interacts with the main field, causing a physical force to be applied to the coil. The electric current is passed through the gradient coils intermittently; each time the current is started or stopped (or changes level), the coils are displaced slightly, but abruptly, producing a sharp sound. Because the gradients must be turned on and off many times per second, a machine-gun-like noise is produced, which in some scanners can reach an 80–90 decibel sound level. This is louder than the noise in an automobile travelling at 100 kilometers per hour with the windows open.

Patient Discomfort

From the subjects' perspective, they are passed through a metal detector and placed on a hard bed. They are then pushed into a narrow tunnel until they come to rest deep inside some mysterious machine. They are told to remain immobile and that there will be a loud noise while they are actually being examined. Although there is voice communication via an intercom to the operator, the patients do not hear anyone in the room with them. After about 15 minutes of this isolation, the machine-gun-like noise stops, and a voice tells them to relax. After perhaps two to three minutes the original instructions are repeated and another 15 minute period of noise is endured. If all has gone well and the scan is satisfactory, they are pulled out of the tunnel and released.

To endure this noisy confinement without moving requires a very cooperative patient with considerable self control. If the patient is in pain, has a short attention span, has obstructed respiration, or any other reason to move, they are not suitable for scanning by current apparatus. This restriction may involve a substantial fraction of hospitalized patients. Undoubtedly, with further hardware and software development, scan times will be substantially shortened and the gradient coil noise muffled.

An X-ray CT scanner, on the other hand, requires immobility in a relatively unconfined space for only 2–10 seconds (for each slice). The CT scanner is almost silent. Almost all patients can be examined for the needed series of these brief scan periods. As with magnetic imaging, there is no patient awareness of the actual interaction of the diagnostic probe with their body.

Pacemakers

A cardiac pacemaker consists of a small electronic package surgically implanted under the skin high on the anterior chest wall, with stimulating wires extending into the subclavian vein and, ultimately, into the apex of the right ventricle. These devices usually are of the demand type, which trigger heart action only after a preset period of electrical silence (a few seconds). They may rarely fire and, to test their viability, a magnetically sensitive switch is included in the device. This switch can be activated by a permanent magnet placed on the skin over the pacemaker, which is turned on to create a preset regular heart rhythm. This is a routine test procedure.

Given this situation, it seems unwise to place a patient with a pacemaker into the main field of an MRI scanner, since this will start the pacemaker's regular rhythm. This probably is harmless in most circumstances, even though the patient may be in a scanner for an hour. Nevertheless, placing the patient in the field tampers with this vital device and, at present, most physicians avoid scanning patients known to have a pacemaker. We have heard informally that several patients with pacemakers have been inadvertently scanned without evident harm. Future pacemakers will probably be made insensitive to external magnetic fields and radio-frequency pulses.

Tissue Metal Artifacts

For magnetic imaging to take place, the magnetic field of the scanner must be highly uniform. Metals imbedded in tissues can present a problem in MRI if they are ferromagnetic; since they are attracted to magnets, they also concentrate and distort the magnetic field. Iron and some types of steel are the most common ferromagnetic materials encountered in MRI.

When a piece of iron-steel appears in the field, it creates two problems. First, it concentrates the main-field magnetic lines of force, causing a regional loss of homogeneity. A piece of steel shrapnel only a few millimeters in diameter may effectively erase the image over several centimeters in all directions. Unlike CT, in which artifacts are confined to only those sections in which the metal lies (adjacent sections are completely unaffected), in MRI a significant regional artifact may be caused by a piece of iron so small as to require radiography to identify its location.

Second, near the opening at either end of the main magnet, there is a rapid convergence of the field, causing very steep gradients. Any ferromagnetic material brought into this region will be forcefully attracted into the magnet. Although this could conceivably be a problem with iron imbedded in the body, it is more often a problem with large objects such as tanks of gas or wrenches. Such objects can be accelerated so abruptly that this has been called the missile effect.

In one case report, an unrecognized small piece of steel in the eye of the patient moved upon entering an MRI scanner, resulting in hemorrhage and visual impairment (Kelly et al., 1986).

Elongated iron structures tend to align themselves with the field and generate a torque, much as a compass needle aligning with the Earth's field. This torque is much stronger than that experienced by a compass needle, however, since the MRI scanner's field can be 20,000–30,000 times stronger than the Earth's field. This could be a source of danger in patients having ferromagnetic clips on blood vessels. Although this has been the subject of much speculation, there has been no published report of injury. This possibility should not be ignored, however; there are many rare clinical complications that remain unpublished, and future clips should not be ferromagnetic.

Fortunately, most metals implanted surgically are not significantly ferromagnetic. All steels are predominately iron, but high nickel content steels (over about 15% nickel) are only weakly ferromagnetic. Dental fillings of mercury-silver amalgam or gold are not at all ferromagnetic. Similarly, tantalum, silver, copper, plastics, lead bullets, and other materials commonly implanted in the body are not ferromagnetic (see reviews by Paul New, 1983). MRI ignores most metals: They appear as voids, as does bone.

Metal detectors (as used in airports) at the entrances of the room housing the scanner magnet now are routine, but they sense only fairly large objects. Vascular clips cannot be detected other than by radiography. When there is any doubt, a radiograph of the patient will establish the presence of tissue metals. It will not, however, determine if they are ferromagnetic.

Complexity and Cost

MRI is the most complex technology yet applied to clinical medicine. Its predecessor, CT scanning, is perhaps an order of magnitude simpler in theory and practice. MRI hardware and physician training are accordingly more expensive. In addition to the interpreting physician, at least two technical operators usually are required.

As noted in Chapter 6, magnetic and electrical shielding are needed for optimal performance. These add to the site costs and tend to limit possible locations. Particularly for high-field machines, this may require locating the site at some inconvenient distance from other related imaging apparatus.

In view of the smaller patient throughput, the much greater cost of purchasing, site preparation, and maintaining the hardware of the MRI scanner, the procedure is accordingly more costly. As currently marketed, with superconductive magnets of high field strength, there is some doubt about MRI's commercial viability.

A substantial reduction of manufacturing cost may result from newer superconducting ceramics, which become superconducting at temperatures above 100° Kelvin. Because this is substantially above the boiling point of nitrogen, liquid nitrogen can be used for cooling. If these ceramics are shown to be practical for use in large MRI magnets, they will greatly simplify the internal structure of the magnets and obviate the need for liquid helium.

CHAPTER 9: THE FUTURE OF MRI

Despite our attempts at simplification, a reader might still conclude that MRI is a very complex process with many interdependent factors. This complexity is both bewildering and a source of hope and challenge. To exploit the magnetic properties of tissues for clinical imaging, MRI scanners, which are probably an order of magnitude more complicated than CT scanners, have been built. However, the complexity of the magnetic properties of tissues offers the possibility of many diagnostic strategies. In the next decade, we can expect changes in both the hardware and the diagnostic strategies employed by the MRI scanner.

SOFTWARE AND PULSE SEQUENCING

As we have stated before, the use of pulse-sequencing in MRI offers many possibilities. The variables that can be adjusted in designing a pulse sequence can be compared to the pieces and moves of a chess game: Because there are many different types of chess men, each with its unique moves, there are many strategies that can be developed in a game of chess. Similarly, in MRI, new pulse sequences are constantly being designed.

Several tissue characteristics already being exploited by MRI are mentioned in Chapter 8: T_1 and T_2 relaxation times, and imaging of moving blood. It is possible that angiography by present invasive means ultimately will be nearly entirely supplanted by MRI; this will apply not only to brain vasculature but to coronary arteries and elsewhere. Regional bone marrow imaging may be developed; recently, regional tissue magnetic susceptibility has been measured.

When considering MRI development, it is important to remember that once the scanner hardware (main magnet, gradient coils, excitation and receiving coils, and a powerful computer) are in place, much developmental work can be done by altering the computer software, to vary pulse sequences, gradient switching, etc. Because this can be accomplished without the need for new hardware, the rate of scanner obsolescence should be slower with MRI than has been the case with CT.

HARDWARE TRENDS — MAIN MAGNETS

For clinical MRI scanners, there probably will be a trend toward much lower field strengths, perhaps generated by permanent magnets. Their low cost, lack of maintenance, small site requirement, and trivial fringe field may find a market in applications where only tissue imaging is required.

The newly announced ceramic superconductors are revolutionary because they are superconductive at relatively high temperatures; they need only be cooled to a temperature approximately 100° above that of liquid helium. They may impact heavily on high-field MRI technology if these brittle substances can be fabricated into a reliable wire.

In the mid-1980s there was a trend toward high-field 1–2 tesla scanners, much of which was justified on the basis of chemical shift spectroscopy, which requires the strongest feasible field. Nuclei other than hydrogen have tissue concentrations many orders of magnitude less than hydrogen and are much less efficient resonators (and produce less signal) than hydrogen. For example, natural fluorine resonates with about 80% of the efficiency of hydrogen; about 23 grams of fluorine in free solution would be required to generate the same signal as one gram of hydrogen.

The success in generating chemical shift spectral peaks of the energetic phosphorus compounds adenosine triphosphate and phosphocreatine (Gadian 1982) has created a misapprehension that clinical chemical shift spectroscopy could have many analytic capabilities.

This is a more difficult problem than might at first be thought. To create sharp spectral peaks, a solute must be in free solution, able to undergo relatively free thermal motion. If the solute is in, or attached to, a membrane or large molecule, it is not freely moving and its T_2 will be shortened because of relatively fixed orientation with other nearby nuclei. This creates large variations in local field strength, and very rapid dephasing.

Many tissue solutes of biological interest are not freely mobile in tissues, while others of little interest are mobile. In brain, for example, the hydrogen spectral peak of water is very much greater than any other. If this peak is sufficiently suppressed (by frequency-selective excitation), other small hydrogen peaks begin to appear. The largest of these is N-acetyl aspartate.

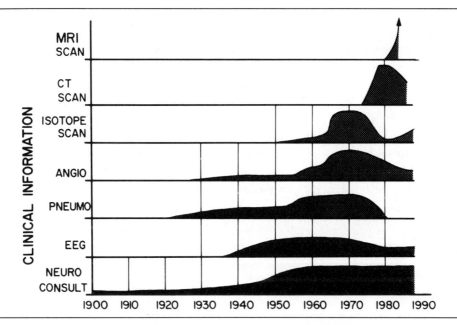

Figure 76. The contribution to neurological patient management of each of several diagnostic modalities 1900–1990 is shown. The introduction of CT in the early 1970s had a significant impact on most of these tests. By the late 1970s, the active development of CT leveled off and subsequently declined. This coincided with increased development of MRI, which has been growing at an exponential rate, indicated by the vertical arrow.

This derivative of aspartic acid has long been recognized as one of the most common small molecules in the brain, but it garnered little interest because it has little, if any, effect on neural activity. If de-acetylated, the residual aspartate is a highly excitatory amino acid. This biological activity of aspartate presumably correlates with some attachment to aspartate receptors imbedded in cell membranes or with incorporation into protein molecules. These attachments would immobilize the aspartate and make it invisible to high resolution spectroscopy. The N-acetyl derivative does not have the alpha–amino acid configuration of natural amino acids, which amino acid receptors need for recognition and attachment, so this derivative probably remains in free solution. The acetyl group would also prevent it from forming peptide bonds to enter into protein synthesis.

One would not choose N-acetyl aspartate as a substance of imaging interest, but it does appear to be mobile in solution. There may well be shown to be some general relationship between the sharpness of NMR spectral peaks and a substance's biological activity. In order to enter into the macromolecule-membrane world of metabolism, a solute may have to anchor itself to some large sluggish structure and, in the process, become invisible to NMR spectroscopy.

CONCLUSIONS

The field of clinical neurology has seen many techniques which harmlessly provided information about the state of the brain's structure (Figure 76).

Although current MRI scanners are masterpieces of engineering and computer science, they undoubtedly are crude by standards that will prevail even a decade from now. The literature in this field has grown enormously in size and diversity since 1980. Many intelligent and resourceful people have recognized the power of MRI in living tissue analysis and imaging.

Modern technology has brought MRI a long way in only a few years. If we could direct to MRI the full force of technology that is now directed toward war and formerly, to exploration of outer space, there seems no limit to what we could learn about our own inner space.

APPENDIX: AN INTRODUCTION TO QUANTUM PROCESS IN MRI

Our observation of the everyday world seems to indicate that processes such as movement and transfer of energy take place smoothly and continuously. However, in the extremely small dimensions of the atom, no continuous processes occur.

Atoms are about one ten-millionth of a millimeter in diameter. A hydrogen nucleus is some 100,000 times smaller. These are too small to be thought of intuitively and can be described only by the abstractions of quantum physics. There are no real-world objects or processes with which to compare the atom and, especially, the much smaller nucleus.

In the world of the atomic nucleus, changes in energy content take place in discrete (quantum) steps rather than as smooth processes. The smoothly changing processes we observe in everyday life are illusions, the result of many smaller discrete quantized processes which, together, make up the familiar processes.

MOTION PICTURES — A QUANTIZED PROCESS
In our childhood, we were all exposed to the movies, in which people and objects moved about apparently as they do in real life. At some time in our development we learned the reality of moving pictures, that the things on the screen are not actually moving, but are only a series of nearly identical pictures flashed on the screen in such rapid succession that they appear to move smoothly. This disillusionment with what our senses tell us is roughly

analogous to the transition from classical Newtonian physics to modern quantum physics.

ENERGY STATES OF THE HYDROGEN NUCLEUS

To describe quantum physics and integrate it with the intricacies of MRI is an exceedingly complex undertaking and beyond the scope of this book. However, as an introduction to the usual literature of MRI, we should describe the alignment, stimulation, and emission of energy for the hydrogen nucleus in the light of modern physics. We will then have a better understanding of the fundamental processes leading to magnetic images, specifically, how the radio signal given off by the nuclei represents nuclear behavior.

ALIGNMENT IN A STRONG MAGNETIC FIELD

When the compass needle aligns itself in the Earth's magnetic field, it comes to rest pointing directly north. In the magnetic field of the MRI scanner, individual hydrogen nuclei attempt to align themselves but cannot align perfectly due to the property of nuclear spin.

In Chapter 2, we saw how the magnetism of certain nuclei results from the property of spin possessed by atomic particles. Nuclear spin cannot be described in terms of rate of rotation or other terms we associate with rotation in the macroscopic world. For example, nuclear spin does not gradually slow down. It is a permanent characteristic of the particle, much as its mass. A useful mechanical analogy to explain how nuclear spin makes the nucleus magnetic describes the nucleus as rotating about an axis. Because the positive charge of the nucleus is located off the axis of rotation, the charge moves in an approximately circular path and produces a magnetic field in a manner analogous to the circulation of electrons in a loop of wire.

The orbiting charge makes the nucleus into a magnet with a north and south pole which lie on its axis of rotation, also called its *spin axis*. The spin axis is represented in diagrams as a straight line passing through the nucleus and extending into space in both directions. Like other magnets, the nucleus will attempt to align itself in a magnetic field so that its south pole seeks the external north pole. (At this point we will note that the end of a compass needle which points at the Earth's north pole is usually marked "North," but is actually the south pole of the magnetized needle). The nucleus does not align perfectly with the field, but tilts away from perfect alignment. The spin axis undergoes a circular wobbling motion more properly termed *precession*. Precessional motion is familiar to us as the motion of a toy top (see Figure 27).

In the above analogies, spin must not be confused with precession. (A toy top in the Earth's gravitational field spins about its axis of rotation at a high rate, but this spin axis precesses at a much slower rate.)

The oscillatory precessional motion of the nucleus in the MRI scanner's magnetic field is comparable to the swinging motion of the compass needle in the Earth's field, described earlier. It can be described by the number of circles of precessional motion the nucleus experiences in one second; this is the larmor (or nuclear magnetic resonant) frequency of the nucleus. The larmor frequency is proportional to the magnetic field strength, and is the frequency at which magnetic energy can be absorbed by the nucleus.

In summary, when the compass needle aligns itself with the Earth's magnetic field, it aligns itself perfectly and comes to rest, the south pole of the compass needle pointing toward the north pole of the Earth. The hydrogen nucleus in the magnetic field of the MRI scanner never comes to rest, but continually precesses. Because of its precessional motion, the south pole of the hydrogen nucleus cannot point directly at the north pole of the external field, but does point in that general direction.

STIMULATION AT THE RESONANT FREQUENCY

The situation described above, with the nucleus precessing and aligned with the field of the scanner, is the low-energy state that the nucleus is in before stimulation. When the hydrogen nucleus is exposed to radio energy at its larmor frequency, the phenomenon of nuclear magnetic resonance occurs: The nucleus absorbs energy.

When it absorbs energy, the nucleus is driven from its resting, or low-energy state into the stimulated, or high-energy state. This corresponds to a change in physical orientation: The nucleus flips in the magnetic field so that its south pole now faces the south pole of the external magnetic field. It continues to precess at its larmor frequency. The nucleus remains in this orientation with some stability, but would "prefer" to return to its low-energy state.

EMISSION OF ENERGY

Having absorbed a quantum of energy, the hydrogen nucleus in watery solutions remains in its high-energy orientation for a period of time ranging up to several seconds, depending on the chemical and physical characteristics of the solution. Eventually, under the influence of the ever-changing magnetic environment of the tissues, the nucleus falls back to its low-energy state. As it does so it re-emits its energy, the lost energy appearing as a radio-frequency photon. The nucleus returns to its original relationship to the magnetic field, its south pole directed toward the external field's north pole (Figure 77).

Whether in its high- or low-energy state, the nucleus precesses at its larmor frequency. The frequency of the emitted photon is the same as the larmor frequency of the nucleus at the moment of decay. If the strength of the magnetic field has been constant throughout the cycle of stimulation and decay, the larmor frequency remains constant, and the emitted photon has the same energy (and frequency) as the original stimulating radio wave. If the

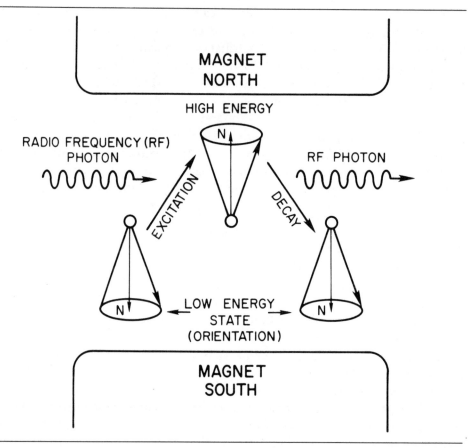

Figure 77. Low- and high-energy orientation. A hydrogen nucleus in its low-energy state (left) absorbs energy from a photon and changes orientation in the field to the high-energy state (center). Subsequently it decays back to the low-energy state (right), giving up energy as a photon.

strength of the magnetic field changes, the photon given off has the new larmor frequency of the nucleus.

HIGH- AND LOW-ENERGY STATES

The stimulation from low- to high-energy states, and subsequent decay from high- to low-energy states, are both quantum processes. The hydrogen nucleus, with its two energy states, is unlike the compass needle, which can be deflected (stimulated) to an infinite number of angles or energy states, depending on how hard it is tapped. (We can note that magnetic nuclei of other elements may occupy several energy states, although still only a limited number.)

A domino lying on a table also has two energy states: lying on one flat side (its low-energy state), and standing on end (its high-energy state). To raise it from horizontal to vertical position, work must be done and energy added.

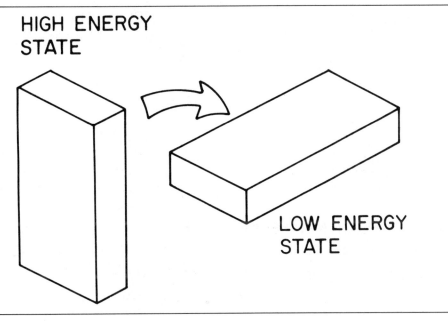

Figure 78. Two energy states of a Domino. A domino standing upright is in its high-energy state. When it falls, it loses energy (as heat and sound) and comes to rest in its low-energy state, lying on its side.

When it is nudged with a horizontal force it falls, giving up (as heat and sound) precisely the amount of energy that it gained on being raised (Figure 78). The raising and falling of the domino is a quantized process, analogous to the stimulation and decay of the hydrogen nucleus, because there are only two states the domino can occupy. The sound given off by the domino is somewhat analogous to the photon emitted when a nucleus falls from a high- to low-energy state.

The difference in energy between the high- and low-energy states of the hydrogen nucleus is precisely the energy of the stimulating radio photon. The frequency of the stimulating photon is that of the larmor frequency of the nucleus, which in turn is related to the field strength. Consequently, the difference between high- and low-energy states is proportional to field strength.

STIMULATED EMISSION
In a further extension of this analogy, consider the horizontal force, or "nudge," required to make the domino fall. Without this force, it would remain forever in its raised, high-energy position. The destabilizing force might come from moving the table randomly until the domino topples. The shaking table is analogous to the random magnetic forces to which an energized nucleus is subjected from thermal motion. These magnetic fluctuations stimulate the emission of energy that determines the rate of energy loss

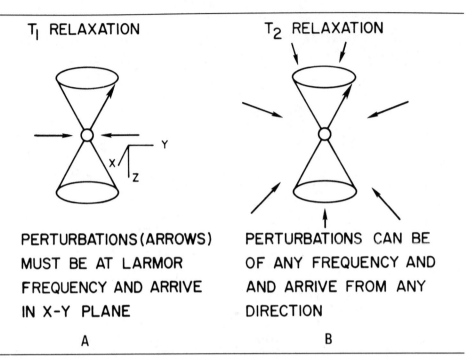

Figure 79. Stimulated emission. Magnetic fluctuations from the tissue environment affect both T_1 and T_2. Fluctuations of any frequency arriving from any direction affect T_2 (B). Only fluctuations at the larmor frequency, arriving perpendicular to the main field, stimulate the emission of energy (T_1) from the nucleus (A).

(T_1). Solids, which lack the random motion of liquids are, by comparison, magnetically very quiet, and so have a very long T_1.

It is the horizontal component of the shaking table which is effective in toppling the domino. In the environment of the tissues, the direction from which the fluctuation arrives is also important: The component of the magnetic fluctuation arriving perpendicular to the main field is most effective at triggering T_1 decay (Figure 79).

CONTINUOUS SIGNAL

One might notice a major discrepancy between the compass needle analogy we originally used as a model for the hydrogen nucleus and the real nucleus we have just described. In our description of the MRI imaging process, we indicated that energy is re-emitted from the tissues in an apparently smooth manner, just as a compass needle loses its energy gradually over a period of seconds, or a bell emits sound over several seconds after being struck. This implied that an individual hydrogen nucleus emits energy in a continuous manner, but as we have just seen, an individual nucleus loses its energy in an instantaneous quantum event, the emission of a weak radio-wave photon.

How can we reconcile the differences between the quantum nature of the

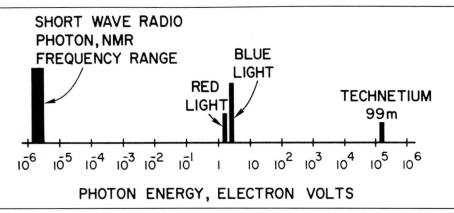

Figure 80. Comparison of photon energy. The energy of the radio photon emitted by the hydrogen nucleus during decay is much less than either visible light or radioactive decay. There are two consequences of this low energy: One is that a very large number of photons is required for the signal to be measurable, the other is that they must be in phase. Visible light, by comparison, need not be in phase in order to be seen, and gamma rays emitted by radioactive decay can be detected individually.

hydrogen nucleus and the observed, seemingly continuous behavior of the free induction decay over several milliseconds? The answer is threefold. First, the radio-wave photon emitted by a single hydrogen nucleus is much too weak to be detected. Second, very large numbers of hydrogen nuclei are involved. Third, the nuclei emit their energy individually over a period of time.

Unlike the photon emitted from radioactive decay of nuclei, radio-wave photons are so weak that only the combined signal of very many photons can be detected by a radio antenna. By contrast, the gamma ray (a photon) emitted by the radioactive decay of one technetium-99m nucleus has an energy of 140,000 electron volts; one such energetic photon can be detected and measured by a gamma ray detector. (For comparison, blue light photons are about three electron volts, red light about two.) (Figure 80).

The energy of the radio-wave photon emitted by one hydrogen nucleus during MRI imaging is approximately one millionth of one electron volt — much too weak to be detected. Any detectable radio signal must consist of the summation of phenomenal numbers of these very low-energy photons. Another consequence of their low energy is that they must be in phase (that is, reinforcing each other) in order to be measurable at all. Visible light need not be in phase in order to be seen, because individual photons are energetic enough to create the molecular changes in our retina necessary for vision.

When tissue is imaged by MRI, trillions of hydrogen nuclei are stimulated into the high-energy state. The largest number of nuclear decays — and thus the strongest signal — occurs immediately after the stimulating radio pulse. As time passes, fewer decays occur and the signal fades.

In summary, although the signal decays in an apparently smooth manner, it is actually made up of many individual, weak radio-frequency photons. The smoothness of the decaying signal is an illusion arising from the large number of nuclei losing their energy.

COMPARISON OF MAGNETIC NUCLEAR DECAY WITH RADIOACTIVE DECAY

In this discussion of the quantum events in MRI, the term *decay* has been used to describe the process in which energy is lost by an individual nucleus. In physics the term decay is most often used to describe radioactive decay, which is instantaneous, and energetic enough to be measured individually. Energetic magnetic decay of a hydrogen nucleus is also instanteous, but the photon it emits is so weak that it cannot be measured individually.

The return to equilibrium of a large population of stimulated hydrogen nuclei over a period of time (milliseconds to hours) is referred to as *relaxation*, rather than decay.

The decay of a hydrogen nucleus which, because of its alignment in a magnetic field, is raised to a high-energy state and subsequently discharges this excess energy as a photon, has several features in common with the decay of certain radioactive isotopes. One familiar type of radioactive decay is that in which a radioactive nucleus — such as carbon-14 — emits a particle and changes its atomic number or weight. In another type of radioactive decay, metastable decay, an energized nucleus emits a photon (a gamma ray) which carries away the excess energy, but the atomic number and weight remain the same.

The most common example is metastable technetium-99 (Tc^{99m}), which is widely used in nuclear medicine. (Technetium does not occur in nature, and all of its isotopes are radioactive. Since it is created artificially, it was named "technetium.") The small "m" after 99 indicates that this nuclide is metastable: It has an excess of energy and is unstable. At some time the nucleus decays, giving up its excess energy as a photon — a gamma ray — which exits the nucleus at the speed of light, leaving it in a much more stable (low-energy) form: Tc^{99}. We can regard the metastable Tc^{99m} to be the high-energy state of the nucleus and the more stable Tc^{99} to be the low-energy form of the nucleus.

After stimulation, the hydrogen nucleus in a magnetic field has several features in common with the Tc^{99m} nucleus: It is in an unstable, high-energy state; it is also destined to undergo decay to a more stable, lower-energy state with the emission of a photon (Figure 81).

But there are major differences between the hydrogen nuclei imaged by MRI and Tc^{99m} decay. First, the photon emitted by the hydrogen nucleus during MRI can have a variable amount of energy, depending on the strength of the scanner's magnetic field. For the Tc^{99m} nucleus, the energy of the emitted photon is always the same — 140,000 electron volts — regardless of

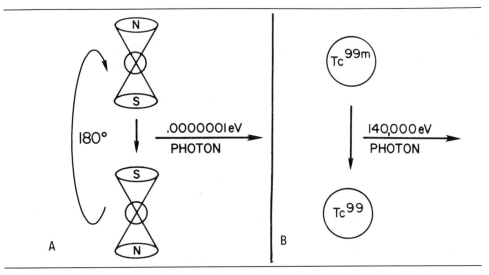

Figure 81A + B. (A) A metastable radioactive nuclide decays from unstable to stable states with emission of a gamma ray without changing its atomic number or weight.
(B) Similarly, a hydrogen nucleus decays from high- to low-energy state with the emission of a radio-frequency photon without changing its nuclear composition.

external conditions. Second, in MRI the rate at which emission of photons takes place varies with the strength of the field, temperature, and chemical environment. In a population of Tc^{99m}, the rate of radioactive decay (half-life) is always the same, regardless of external conditions.

COMPARISON BETWEEN RADIOACTIVE HALF-LIFE AND T_1

A further useful comparison between radioactive nuclei and hydrogen nuclei is in the terminology used to describe the rate at which they emit energy. In MRI, we have seen that as time passes, there are fewer and fewer high-energy nuclei remaining to emit their energy: The strongest signal from the tissues is received immediately after stimulation; after that the number of decays decreases exponentially. The rate of decay of radioactive nuclei such as Tc^{99m} similarly decreases exponentially with time.

The term used to describe the rate of decay of radioactive elements is *half-life*, which is the time it takes one half of the remaining nuclei to decay from their high- to low-energy states. Similarly, the rate at which hydrogen nuclei emit their energy after stimulation is described by the term T_1, which (for mathematical reasons) is defined as the time it takes 63% $(1-1/e)$ of the stimulated hydrogen nuclei to emit their energy. While the half-life of Tc^{99m} under all circumstances is six hours, the T_1 of hydrogen in water is variable, from milliseconds to hours, depending on its chemical and physical composition.

Decay of Tc^{99m} is independent of its chemical or physical environment:

Some circumstance inside the nucleus triggers its decay. No means of changing it is known. T_1 decay must be stimulated by magnetic fluctuations from the external environment (from the lattice). (See discussion on stimulated emission earlier in the Appendix.)

BIBLIOGRAPHY

BOOKS

Bradley, W.G., Adey, W.R., and Hasso, A.N. *Magnetic Resonance Imaging of the Brain, Head, and Neck.* Aspen Systems, Rockville, Maryland, 1985.

Fawcett, D.W. *The Cell.* W.B. Saunders, Philadelphia, PA, 1981.

Farrar, T.C., and Becker, E.D. *Pulse and Fourier Transform NMR.* Academic Press, New York, 1971.

Fukushima, E., and Roeder, S.B. *Experimental Pulse NMR.* Addison-Wesley, Reading, Massachusetts, 1981.

Gadian, D.G. *Nuclear Magnetic Resonance and its Applications to Living Systems.* Clarendon Press, Oxford, 1982.

Kaufman, L., Crooks, L., Margulis, A., Eds. *Nuclear Magnetic Resonance Imaging in Medicine.* Igaku-Shoin, New York, Tokyo, 1981.

Kemp, W. *NMR in Chemistry: A Multinuclear Approach.* Macmillan, London, 1986.

Mansfied, P., and Morris, P.G. *NMR Imaging in Biomedicine.* Academic Press, New York, 1982.

Martin, M.L., Martin, G.J., and Delpeuch, J. *Practical NMR Spectroscopy.* Heyden and Son, London, 1980.

Oldendorf, W.H. *The Quest for an Image of Brain.* Raven Press, New York, 1980.

Pagels, Heinz R., *The Cosmic Code: Quantum Physics as the Language of Nature.* Pelican, Middlesex, 1984.

Partain, C.L., Price, Patton, Kulkarni, and James, Eds. *Magnetic Resonance (MR) Imaging.* Second edition. W.B. Saunders, 1987.

Valk, J., Maclean, C., and Algra, P.R. *Basic Principles of Nuclear Magnetic Resonance Imaging.* Elsevier, Amsterdam, New York, Oxford, 1985.

Young, S.W. *Nuclear Magnetic Resonance Imaging: Basic Principles.* Raven Press, New York, 1984.

ARTICLES

Bloch, F., Hanson, W., and Packard, M. "Nuclear induction." *Phys. Rev.* **69**: 127, 1946.

Bore, P.J., Galloway, G.J., Styles, P., Radda, G.K., Flynn, G., and Pitts, P.R. "Are quenches dangerous?" *Magnetic Resonance in Medicine* **3**: 112–117, 1986.

Bottomley, P.A., Foster, T.H., Argersinger, R.E., and Pfeifer, L.M. "A review of normal tissue hydrogen NMR relaxation times and relaxation mechanisms from 1–100 MHz: Dependence on tissue type, NMR frequency, temperature, species, excision and age." *Med. Phys.* **11**: 425–448, 1984.

Kelly, W.M., Paglen, P.G., Pearson, J.A., San Diego, A.G., and Soloman, M.A. "Ferromagnetism of intraocular foreign body causes unilateral blindness after MR study." *AJNR* **7**: 243–245, 1986.

Lauterbur, P.C., "Image formation by induced local interactions: Examples employing nuclear magnetic resonance." *Nature* **242**: 5394: 190, 1973.

New, P.F., Rosen, B.R., Brady, T.J., Buonanno, F.S., Kistler, J.P., Burt, C.T., Hinshaw, W.S., Newhouse, J.H., Pohost, G.M., and Taveras, J.M. "Potential hazards and artifacts of ferromagnetic and nonferromagnetic surgical and dental materials and devices in nuclear magnetic resonance." *Radiology* **147**: 139–148, 1983.

Purcell, E., Torrey, H., and Pound, R. "Resonance absorption by nuclear magnetic moments in a solid." *Phys. Rev.* **69**: 37–38, 1946.

INDEX

Aluminum, use in resistive coils 93–4
Artifacts
   tissue metal artifacts in CT 120–121
   tissue metal artifacts in MRI 136–137
   from movement 123
Autopsy, effect of CT on 6
Axis of rotation, *see spin axis*

Background noise, *see signal-to-noise ratio*
Blood
   moving, visualized by MRI 128–130,
     139
   stagnant, visualization by MRI 45
Blood-brain barrier, defects in 117–118
Bloch, Felix 66
Bone
   appearance in CT 115
   appearance in MRI 115, 125–126
   comparison CT and MRI 29
Bone marrow, possible regional studies
   129, 139
Brownian motion 36
Building modifications in MRI — *see site
   preparation*

Ceramic superconducting magnets, *see high-
   temperature superconducting magnets*
Cerebrospinal fluid
   T-one and T-two of 82
   tidal movements, visualized in MRI
     129
Chelates in MRI contrast media 131
Chemical shift spectral analyzers 101, 106
Chemical shift spectroscopy in MRI 104,
   140, 101
Claustrophobia, *see patient confinement*
Compact bone *see bone*
Compass needle
   magnetic properties 7–10
   natural frequency 7
Components of MRI scanner 89
Computer reconstruction in MRI 26–27
   comparison of CT and MRI 28–29
   Fourier transform 27
Computerized tomography (CT)
   evolution of design 121–122
   invention of 3
   limitations of 115, 123
   future of 123
   contributions of 3–5, 123